Anti-Inflammatory Breakfast Recipe Book

A varied collection of recipes for your anti inflammatory diet

Natalie Worley

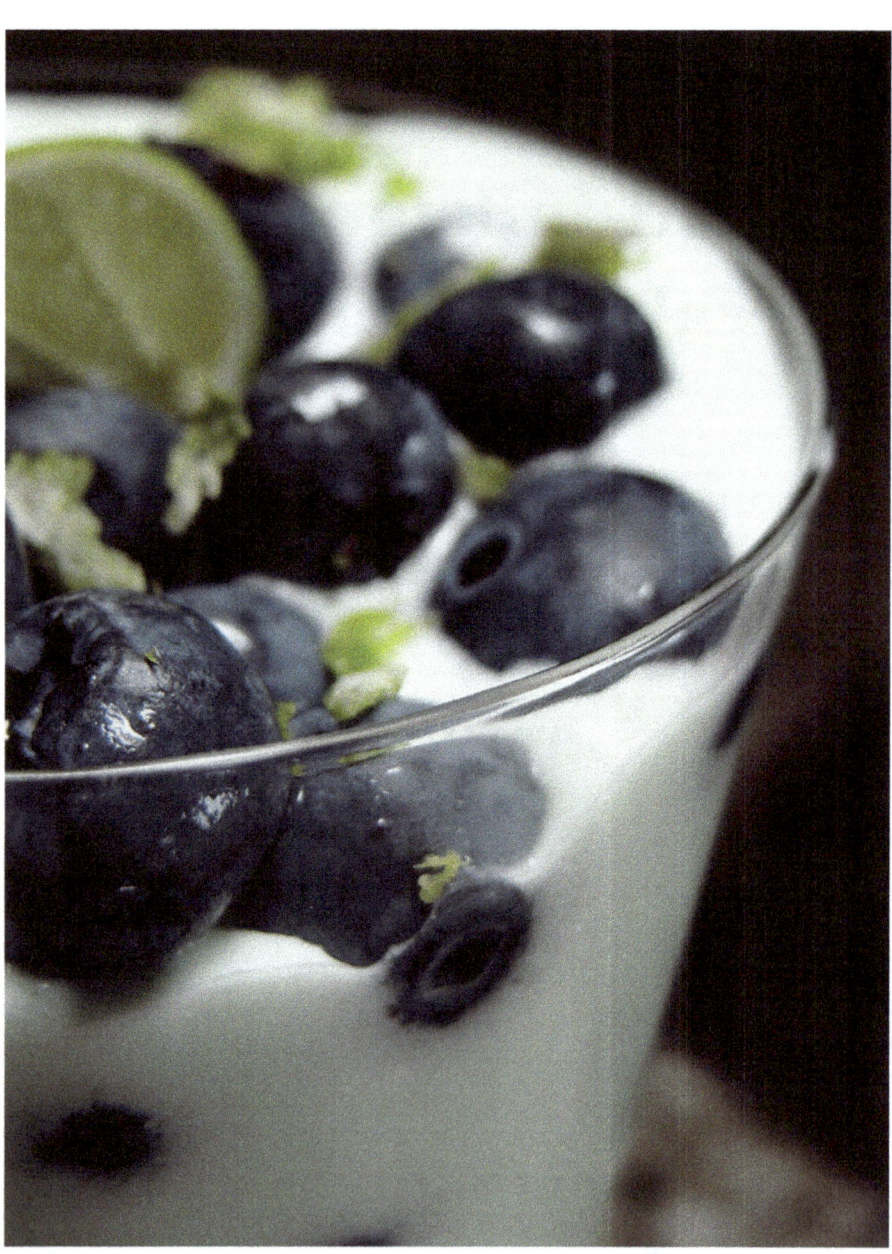

© copyright 2021 – all rights reserved.

the content contained within this book may not be reproduced, duplicated or transmitted without direct written permission from the author or the publisher.

under no circumstances will any blame or legal responsibility be held against the publisher, or author, for any damages, reparation, or monetary loss due to the information contained within this book. either directly or indirectly.

legal notice:

this book is copyright protected. this book is only for personal use. you cannot amend, distribute, sell, use, quote or paraphrase any part, or the content within this book, without the consent of the author or publisher.

disclaimer notice:

please note the information contained within this document is for educational and entertainment purposes only. all effort has been executed to present accurate, up to date, and reliable, complete information. no warranties of any kind are declared or implied. readers acknowledge that the author is not engaging in the rendering of legal, financial, medical or professional advice. the content within this book has been derived from various sources. please consult a licensed professional before attempting any techniques outlined in this book.

by reading this document, the reader agrees that under no circumstances is the author responsible for any losses, direct or indirect, which are incurred as a result of the use of information contained within this document, including, but not limited to, — errors, omissions, or inaccuracies.

Table of Contents

- BLACKBERRIES BOWLS 7
- CILANTRO OMELET 8
- TOMATOES AND SWISS CHARD BAKE 10
- PUMPKIN SPICE MUFFINS 12
- STRAWBERRIES OATMEAL 15
- TUNA AND SPRING ONIONS SALAD 17
- SCRAMBLED EGGS 19
- HERBED EGGS 20
- CHERRY TOMATOES OMELET 22
- BASIL EGGS 24
- ZUCCHINI AND ARTICHOKES MIX 25
- PAPRIKA EGGS AND BROCCOLI 27
- RASPBERRIES OATMEAL 28
- ZUCCHINI SPREAD 30
- BREAKFAST KALE FRITTATA 32
- CRANBERRY GRANOLA BARS 33
- SPINACH AND BERRY SMOOTHIE 34
- ZUCCHINI BREAKFAST SALAD 36
- QUINOA AND SPINACH BREAKFAST SALAD 37
- CARROTS BREAKFAST MIX 38
- ITALIAN BREAKFAST SALAD 41

Zucchini and Sprout Breakfast Mix	44
Breakfast Corn Salad	45
Simple Basil Tomato Mix	46
Cucumber and Avocado Salad	47
Watermelon Salad	49
Prep Time: 10 min	Cook Time: 0 min	Serve: 2	49
Peppers and Olives Salad	51
Sweet Potato, Spinach, and Eggs Mix	53
Avocado and Mango Salad	55
Brussels Sprouts Eggs with Turmeric	57
Strawberries and Spinach Bowls	59
Collard and Spinach Oatmeal	60
Spinach, Kale and Quinoa Salad	63
Fennel, Kale and Barley Salad	65
Chili Carrot and Sweet Potato Mix	67
Jalapeno Cucumber Bowls	70
Zucchinis, Arugula, and Barley Mix	72
Avocado and Pepper Eggs Mix	74
Olives Frittata with Shallots	77
Berries Coconut Mix	79
Cucumber, Spinach, and Olives Salad	80
Sweet Potato Bowls	83

SHALLOTS CUCUMBER OMELET 85
CINNAMON OATMEAL WITH MAPLE SYRUP 88
CHILI BROCCOLI SALAD 91
SPINACH, KALE, AND OLIVES BOWLS 94
CHERRY TOMATO AND ORANGE SALAD 97
PEAR AND KALE SALAD 100
BERRIES AND CANTALOUPE SALAD 101
CAULIFLOWER AND EGGS MIX 103

Blackberries Bowls

Prep Time: 20 minutes | **Serve:** 4

- 1 ½ cups coconut milk
- ½ cup coconut; shredded
- ½ cup blackberries
- 2 tsp. stevia

1. In your air fryer's pan, mix all the ingredients, stir, cover and cook at 360°F for 15 minutes.

Nutrition: Calories: 171; Fat: 4g; Fiber: 2g; Carbs: 3g; Protein: 5g

Cilantro Omelet

Prep Time: 25 minutes | **Serve:** 4

- 6 eggs; whisked
- 1 cup mozzarella; shredded
- 1 cup cilantro; chopped.
- Cooking spray
- Salt and black pepper to taste.

1.Take a bowl and mix all the ingredients except the cooking spray and whisk well.
2.Grease a pan that fits your air fryer with the cooking spray, pour the eggs mix, spread, put the pan into the machine, and cook at 350°F for 20 minutes
3.Divide the omelet between plates and serve for breakfast.

Nutrition: Calories: 270; Fat: 15g; Fiber: 3g; Carbs: 5g; Protein: 9g

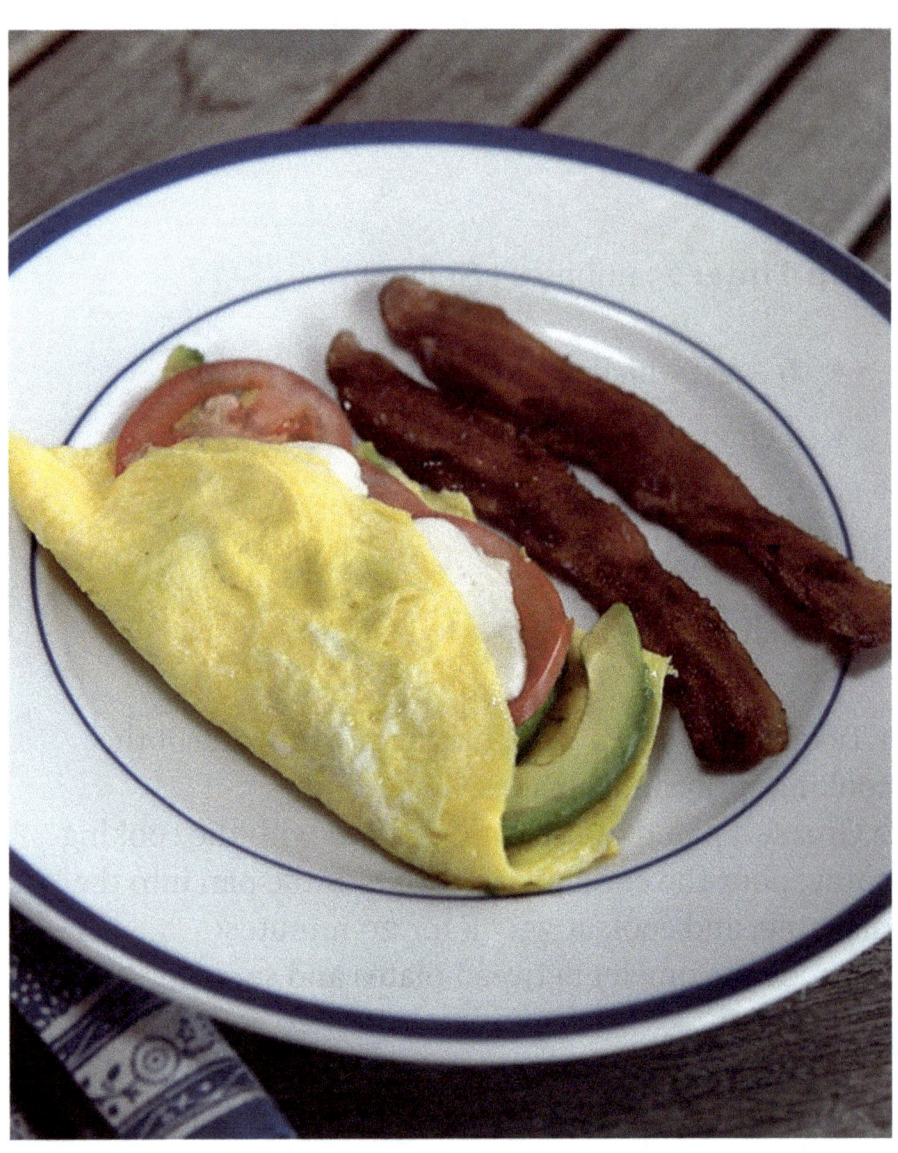

Tomatoes and Swiss Chard Bake

Prep Time: 20 minutes | **Serve:** 4

- 4 eggs; whisked
- 3 oz. Swiss chard; chopped.
- 1 cup tomatoes; cubed
- 1 tsp. olive oil
- Salt and black pepper to taste.

1. Take a bowl and mix the eggs with the rest of the ingredients except the oil and whisk well.
2. Grease a pan that fits the fryer with the oil, pour the swiss chard mix and cook at 359°F for 15 minutes.

Nutrition: Calories: 202; Fat: 14g; Fiber: 3g; Carbs: 5g; Protein: 12g

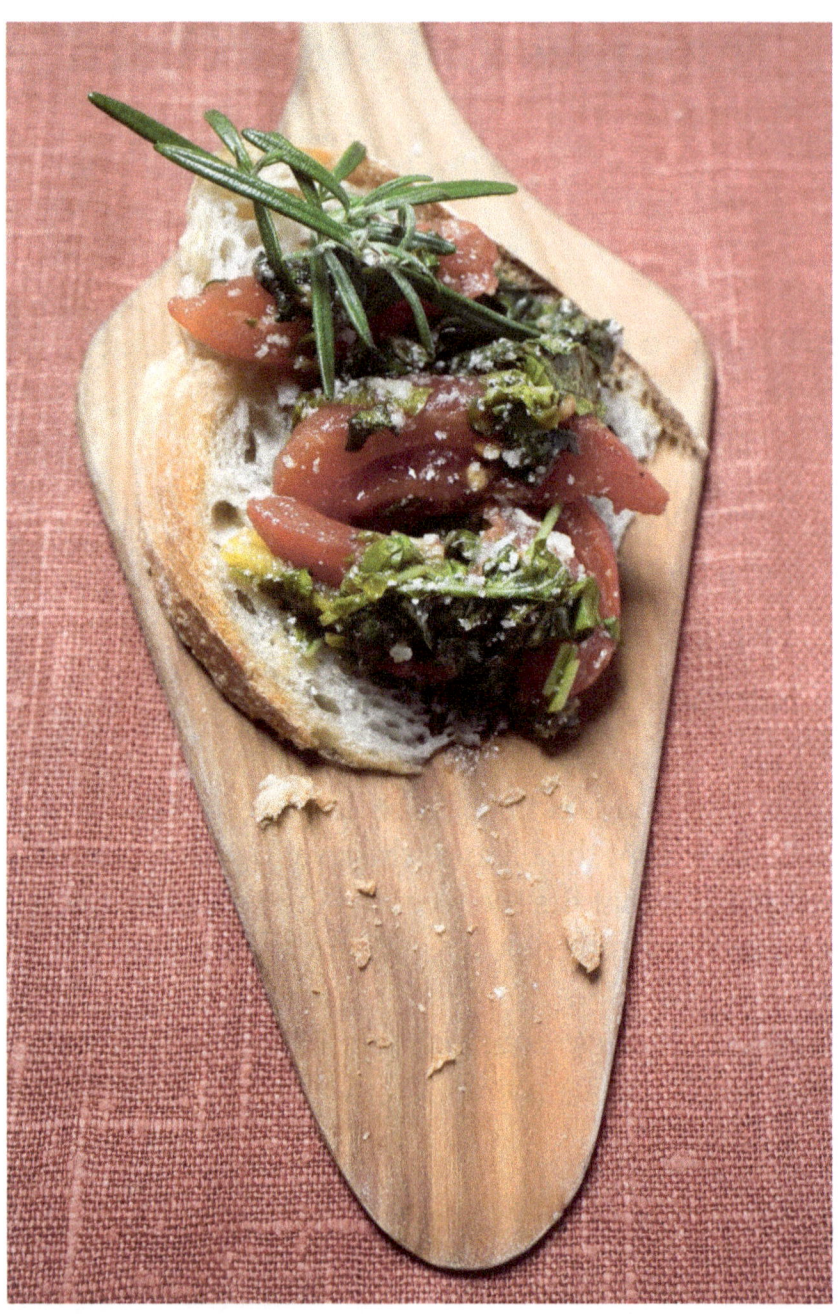

Pumpkin Spice Muffins

Prep Time: 25 minutes | **Serve:** 6

- 2 large eggs.
- 1 cup blanched finely ground almond flour.
- ¼ cup unsalted butter; softened.
- ¼ cup pure pumpkin purée.
- ½ cup granular erythritol. ¼ tsp. Ground nutmeg.
- 1 tsp. vanilla extract.
- ½ tsp. ground cinnamon.
- ½ tsp. Baking powder.

1.Take a large bowl, mix almond flour, erythritol, baking powder, butter, pumpkin purée, cinnamon, nutmeg, and vanilla. Gently stir in eggs.
2.Evenly pour the batter into six silicone muffin cups. Place muffin cups into the air fryer basket, working in batches if necessary.
3.Adjust the temperature to 300 Degrees F and set the timer for 15 minutes. When completely cooked, a toothpick inserted in the center will come out mostly clean. Serve warm.

Nutrition: Calories: 205; Protein: 6.3g; Fiber: 2.4g; Fat: 18.0g; Carbs: 17.4g

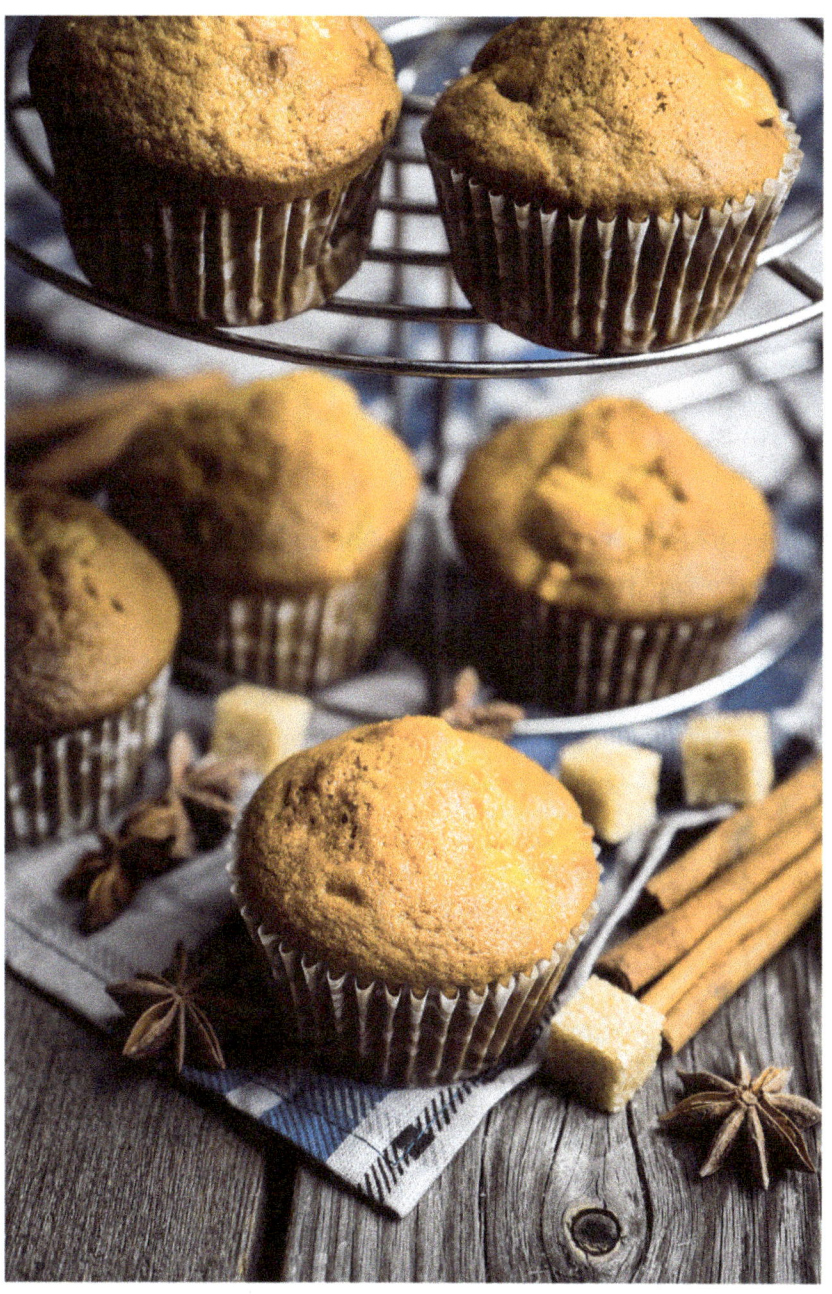

Strawberries Oatmeal

Prep Time: 20 minutes | **Serve:** 4

- ½ cup coconut; shredded ¼ cup strawberries
- 2 cups coconut milk ¼ tsp. vanilla extract 2 tsp. stevia Cooking spray

1.Grease the Air Fryer's pan with the cooking spray, add all the ingredients inside, and toss
2.Cook at 365°F for 15 minutes, divide into bowls and serve for breakfast.

Nutrition: Calories: 142; Fat: 7g; Fiber: 2g; Carbs: 3g; Protein: 5g

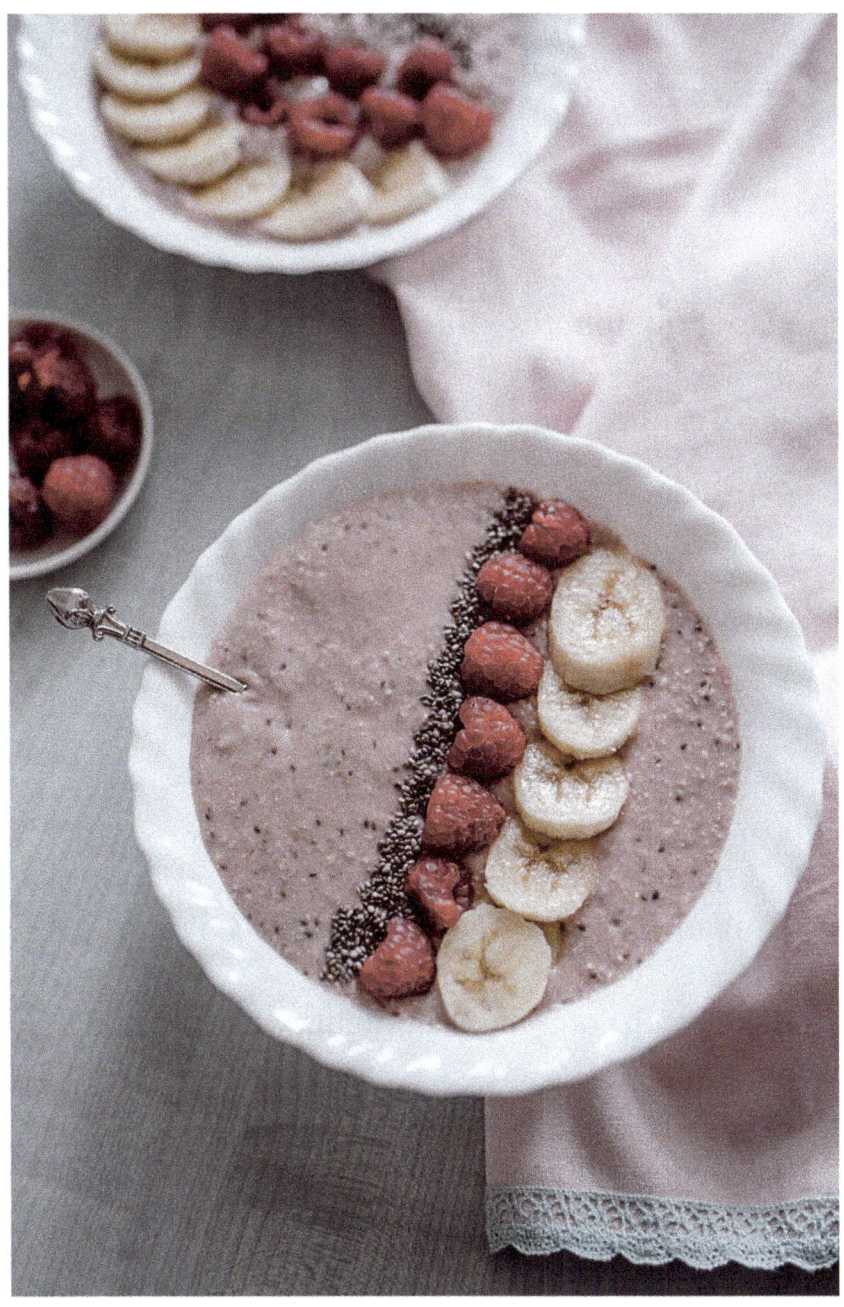

Tuna and Spring Onions Salad

Prep Time: 20 minutes | **Serve:** 4

- 14 oz. canned tuna drained and flaked
- 2 spring onions; chopped.
- 1 cup arugula
- 1 tbsp. olive oil
- A pinch of salt and black pepper

1. In a bowl, all the ingredients except the oil and the arugula and whisk.
2. Preheat the Air Fryer over 360°F, add the oil, and grease it. Pour the tuna mix, stir well and cook for 15 minutes
3. In a salad bowl, combine the arugula with the tuna mix, toss and serve.

Nutrition: Calories: 212; Fat: 8g; Fiber: 3g; Carbs: 5g; Protein: 8g

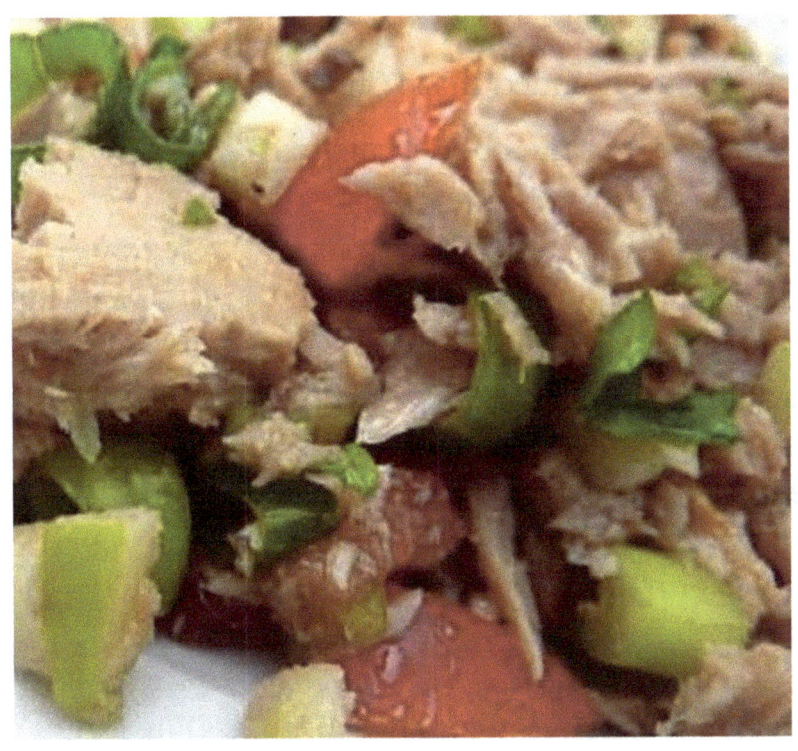

Scrambled Eggs

Prep Time: 20 minutes | **Serve:** 2

- 4 large eggs.
- ½ cup shredded sharp Cheddar cheese.
- 2 tbsp. unsalted butter; melted.

1. Crack eggs into a 2-cup round baking dish and whisk. Place dish into the air fryer basket.
2. Adjust the temperature to 400 Degrees F and set the timer for 10 minutes
3. After 5 minutes, stir the eggs and add the butter and cheese. Let cook 3 more minutes and stir again
4. Allow eggs to finish cooking for an additional 2 minutes or remove if they are to your desired liking. Use a fork to fluff.

Nutrition: Calories: 359; Protein: 19.5g; Fiber: 0.0g; Fat: 27.6g; Carbs: 1.1g

Herbed Eggs

Prep Time: 25 minutes | **Serve:** 4

- ½ cup cheddar; shredded
- 10 eggs; whisked
- 2 tbsp. chives; chopped.
- 2 tbsp. basil; chopped.
- 2 tbsp. parsley; chopped. Cooking spray
- Salt and black pepper to taste.

1.Take a bowl and mix the eggs with all the ingredients except the cheese and the cooking spray and whisk well
2.Preheat the air fryer at 350°F, grease it with the cooking spray, and pour the eggs mixture inside
3.Sprinkle the cheese on top and cook for 20 minutes. Divide everything between plates and serve.

Nutrition: Calories: 232; Fat: 12g; Fiber: 4g; Carbs: 5g; Protein: 7g

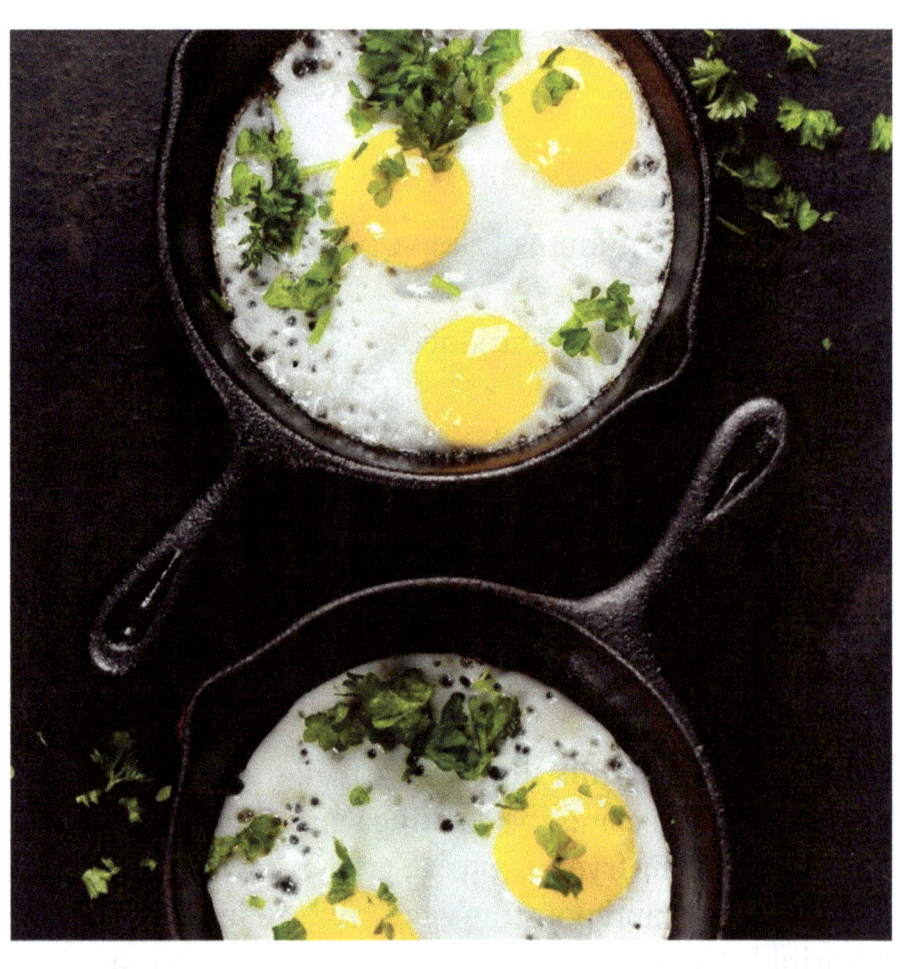

Cherry Tomatoes Omelet

Prep Time: 25 minutes | **Serve:** 4

- 1 lb. cherry tomatoes; halved
- 4 eggs; whisked
- 1 tbsp. cheddar; grated
- 1 tbsp. parsley; chopped.
- Salt and black pepper to taste.
- Cooking spray

1.Put the tomatoes in the air fryer's basket, cook at 360°F for 5 minutes and transfer them to the baking pan that fits the machine greased with cooking spray
2.Take a bowl, mix the eggs with the remaining ingredients, whisk, pour over the tomatoes, and cook at 360°F for 15 minutes.

Nutrition: Calories: 230; Fat: 14g; Fiber: 3g; Carbs: 5g; Protein: 11g

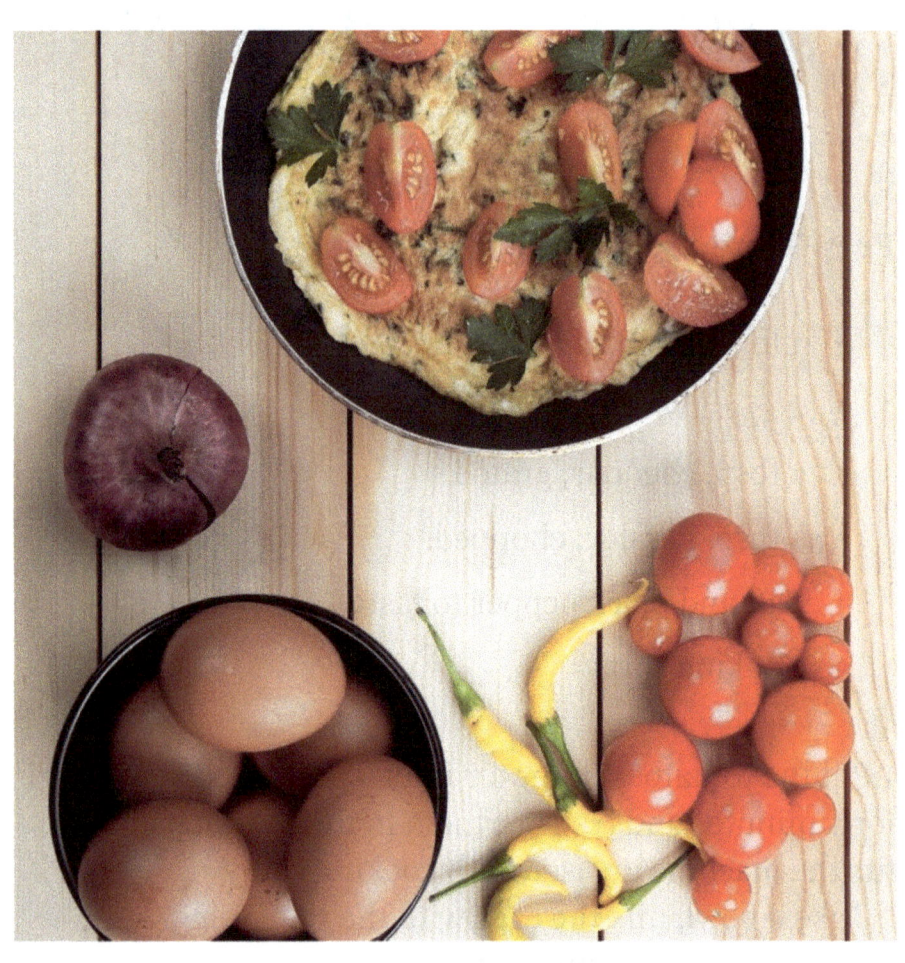

Basil Eggs

Prep Time: 25 minutes | **Serve:** 4

- 1 cup mozzarella cheese; grated
- 6 eggs; whisked
- 2 tbsp. basil; chopped.
- 2 tbsp. butter; melted
- 6 tsp. basil pesto
- A pinch of salt and black pepper

1. Take a bowl and mix all the ingredients except the butter and whisk them well.
2. Preheat your Air Fryer at 360°F, drizzle the butter on the bottom, spread the eggs mix, cook for 20 minutes and serve for breakfast

Nutrition: Calories: 207; Fat: 14g; Fiber: 3g; Carbs: 4g; Protein: 8g

Zucchini and Artichokes Mix

Prep Time: 25 minutes | **Serve:** 4

- 8 oz. canned artichokes, drained and chopped.
- 2 tomatoes; cut into quarters
- 4 eggs; whisked
- 4 spring onions; chopped.
- 2 zucchinis; sliced
- Cooking spray
- Salt and black pepper to taste.

1.Grease a pan with cooking spray and mix all the other ingredients inside.
2.Put the pan in the Air Fryer and cook at 350°F for 20 minutes. Divide between plates and serve

Nutrition: Calories: 210; Fat: 11g; Fiber: 3g; Carbs: 4g; Protein: 6g

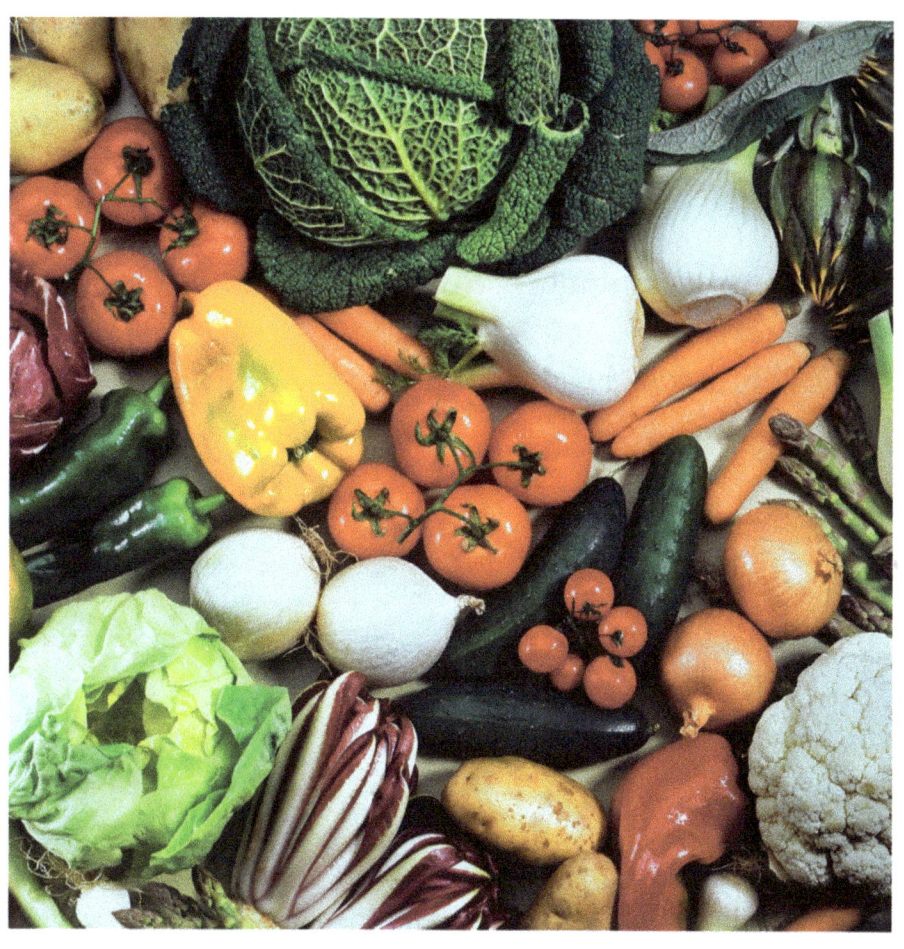

Paprika Eggs and Broccoli

Prep Time: 25 minutes | **Serve:** 4

- 1 broccoli head, florets separated and roughly chopped.
- 4 oz. sour cream
- Cooking spray
- 2 eggs; whisked
- Salt and black pepper to taste.
- 1 tbsp. sweet paprika

1.Grease a pan that fits your air fryer with the cooking spray and mix all the ingredients inside.
2.Put the pan in the Air Fryer and cook at 360°F for 20 minutes. Divide between plates and serve

Nutrition: Calories: 220; Fat: 14g; Fiber: 2g; Carbs: 3g; Protein: 2g

Raspberries Oatmeal

Prep Time: 20 minutes | **Serve:** 4

- 1 ½ cups coconut; shredded
- ½ cups raspberries
- 2 cups almond milk ¼ tsp. Nutmeg ground 2 tsp. stevia
- ½ tsp. cinnamon powder Cooking spray

1.Grease the air fryer's pan with cooking spray, mix all the ingredients inside, cover and cook at 360°F for 15 minutes.

Nutrition: Calories: 172; Fat: 5g; Fiber: 2g; Carbs: 4g; Protein: 6g

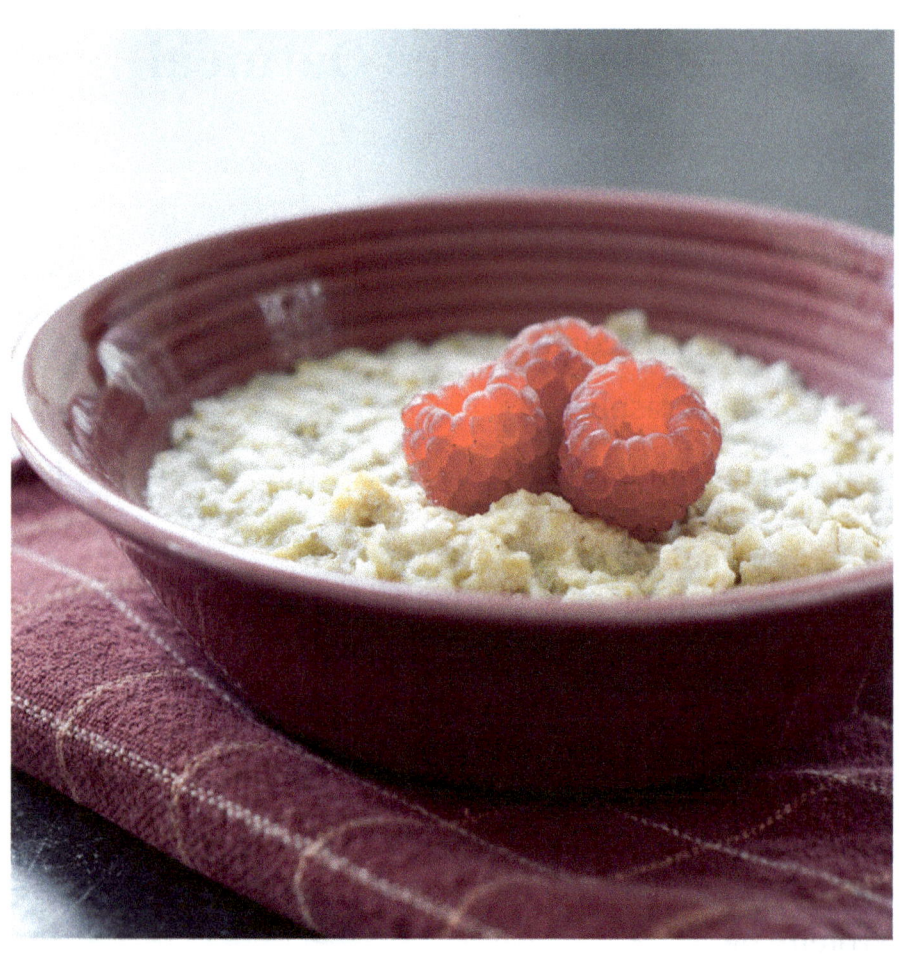

Zucchini Spread

Prep Time: 20 minutes | **Serve:** 4

- 4 zucchinis; roughly chopped.
- 1 tbsp. butter; melted
- 1 tbsp. sweet paprika
- Salt and black pepper to taste.

Grease a baking pan that fits the Air Fryer with the butter, add all the ingredients, toss and cook at 360°F for 15 minutes
Transfer to a blender, pulse well, divide into bowls and serve for breakfast.

Nutrition: Calories: 240; Fat: 14g; Fiber: 2g; Carbs: 5g; Protein: 11g

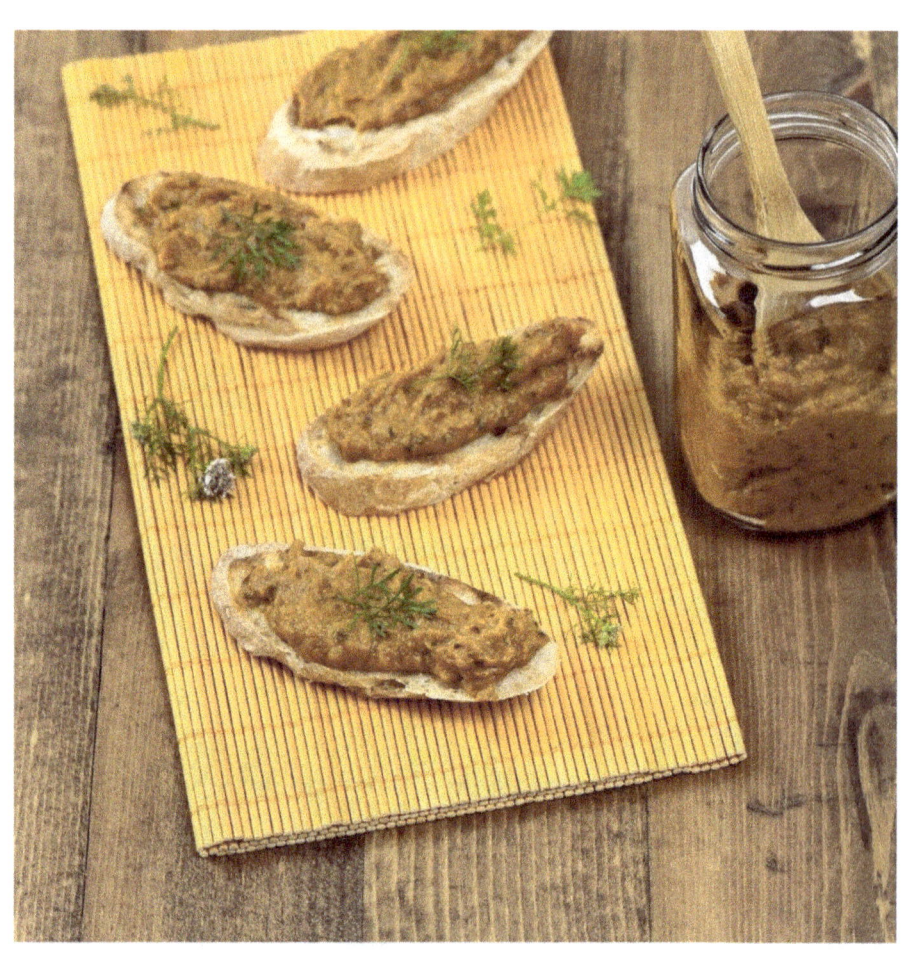

Breakfast Kale Frittata

Prep Time: 10 min | **Cook Time:** 30 min | **Serve:** 4

- 6 kale stalks, chopped
- 1 small sweet onion, chopped
- 1 small broccoli head, florets separated
- 2 garlic cloves, minced
- Salt and black pepper to the taste
- 4 eggs
- 1 tablespoon olive oil

1.Heat a pan with the oil over medium-high heat, add the onion, stir and cook for 4-5 minutes. Add the garlic, broccoli, and kale, toss, and cook for 5 minutes more. Add the eggs, salt, and pepper and mix. Place in the oven and bake at 380 degrees F for 20 minutes. Slice and serve for breakfast.

Nutrition: calories 214, fat 7, fiber 2, carbs 12, protein 8 13.

Cranberry Granola Bars

Prep Time: 2 h | **Cook Time:** 0 min | **Serve:** 4

- 2 cups walnuts, toasted
- 1 cup dates, pitted
- 3 tablespoons water
- ¾ cup cranberries, dried, no added sugar 2 cups desiccated coconut, unsweetened

1.In your food processor, mix dates with coconut, cranberries, water, and walnuts. Pulse well, then spread the mix into a lined baking dish. Press well into the dish and keep in the fridge for 2 hours, then cut into bars and serve.

Nutrition: calories 476, fat 40, fiber 9, carbs 33, protein 6

Spinach and Berry Smoothie

Prep Time: 10 min | **Cook Time:** 0 min | **Serve:** 2

- 1 cup blackberries
- 1 avocado, pitted, peeled, and chopped
- 1 banana, peeled and roughly chopped
- 1 cup baby spinach
- 1 tablespoon hemp seeds
- 1 cup water
- ½ cup almond milk, unsweetened

1.In your blender, mix the berries with the avocado, banana, spinach, hemp seeds, water, and almond milk. Pulse well, divide into 2 glasses, and serve for breakfast.

Nutrition: calories 160, fat 3, fiber 4, carbs 6, protein 3 15.

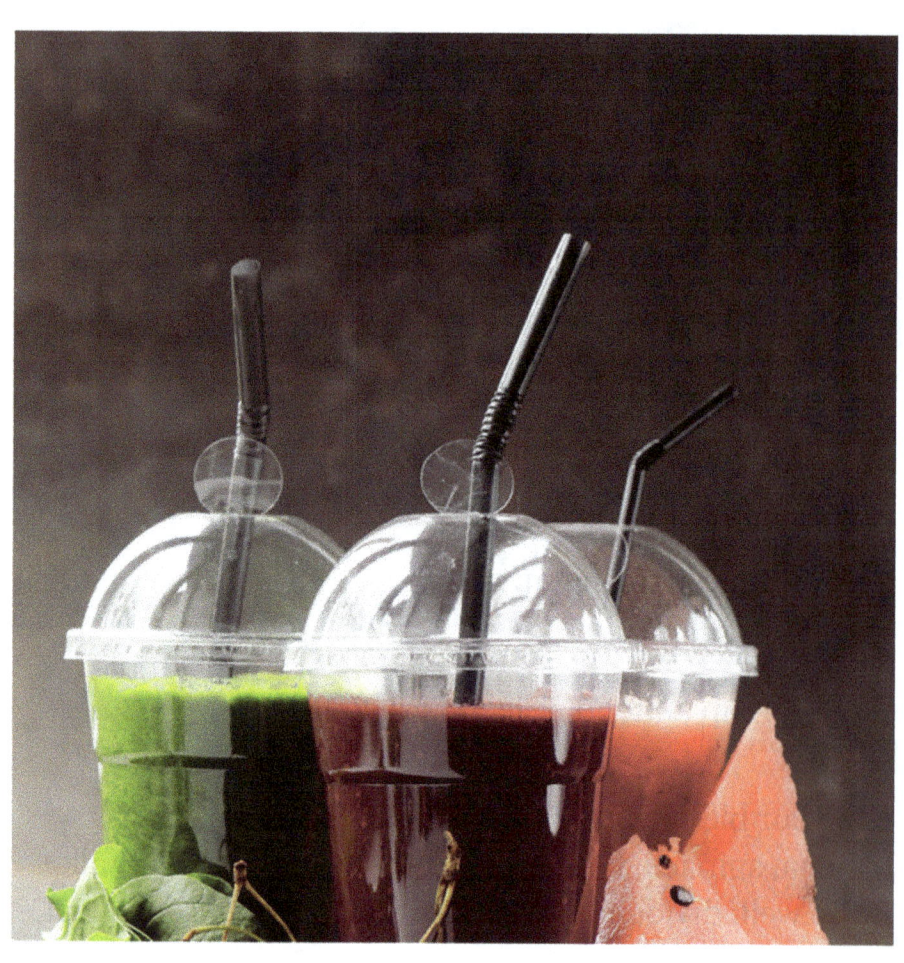

Zucchini Breakfast Salad

Prep Time: 10 min | **Cook Time:** 0 min | **Serve:** 4

- 2 zucchinis, spiralized
- 1 cup beets, baked, peeled, and grated
- ½ bunch kale, chopped
- 2 tablespoons olive oil

For the tahini sauce:
- 1 tablespoon maple syrup
- Juice of 1 lime
- ¼ inch fresh ginger, grated
- 1/3 cup sesame seed paste

1.In a salad bowl, mix the zucchinis with the beets, kale, and oil. In another small bowl, whisk the maple syrup with lime juice, ginger, and sesame paste. Pour the dressing over the salad, toss and serve it for breakfast.

Nutrition: calories 183, fat 3, fiber 2, carbs 7, protein 9 16.

Quinoa and Spinach Breakfast Salad

Prep Time: 10 min | **Cook Time:** 0 min | **Serve:** 2

- 16 ounces quinoa, cooked
- 1 handful raisins
- 1 handful baby spinach leaves
- 1 tablespoon maple syrup
- ½ tablespoon lemon juice
- 4 tablespoons olive oil
- 1 teaspoon ground cumin
- A pinch of sea salt and black pepper
- ½ teaspoon chili flakes

1.In a bowl, mix the quinoa with spinach, raisins, cumin, salt, pepper, and toss. Add the maple syrup, lemon juice, oil, and chili flakes and toss, then serve for breakfast.

Nutrition: calories 170, fat 3, fiber 6, carbs 8, protein 5 17.

Carrots Breakfast Mix

Prep Time: 10 min | **Cook Time:** 0 min | **Serve:** 4

- 1½ tablespoon maple syrup
- 1 teaspoon olive oil
- 1 tablespoon chopped walnuts
- 1 onion, chopped
- 4 cups shredded carrots
- 1 tablespoon curry powder
- ¼ teaspoon ground turmeric
- Black pepper to the taste
- 2 tablespoons sesame seed paste
- ¼ cup lemon juice
- ½ cup chopped parsley

1.In a salad bowl, mix the onion with the carrots, turmeric, curry powder, black pepper, lemon juice, and parsley. Add the maple syrup, oil, walnuts, and sesame seed paste. toss well and serve for breakfast.

Nutrition: calories 150, fat 3, fiber 2, carbs 6, protein 8 18.

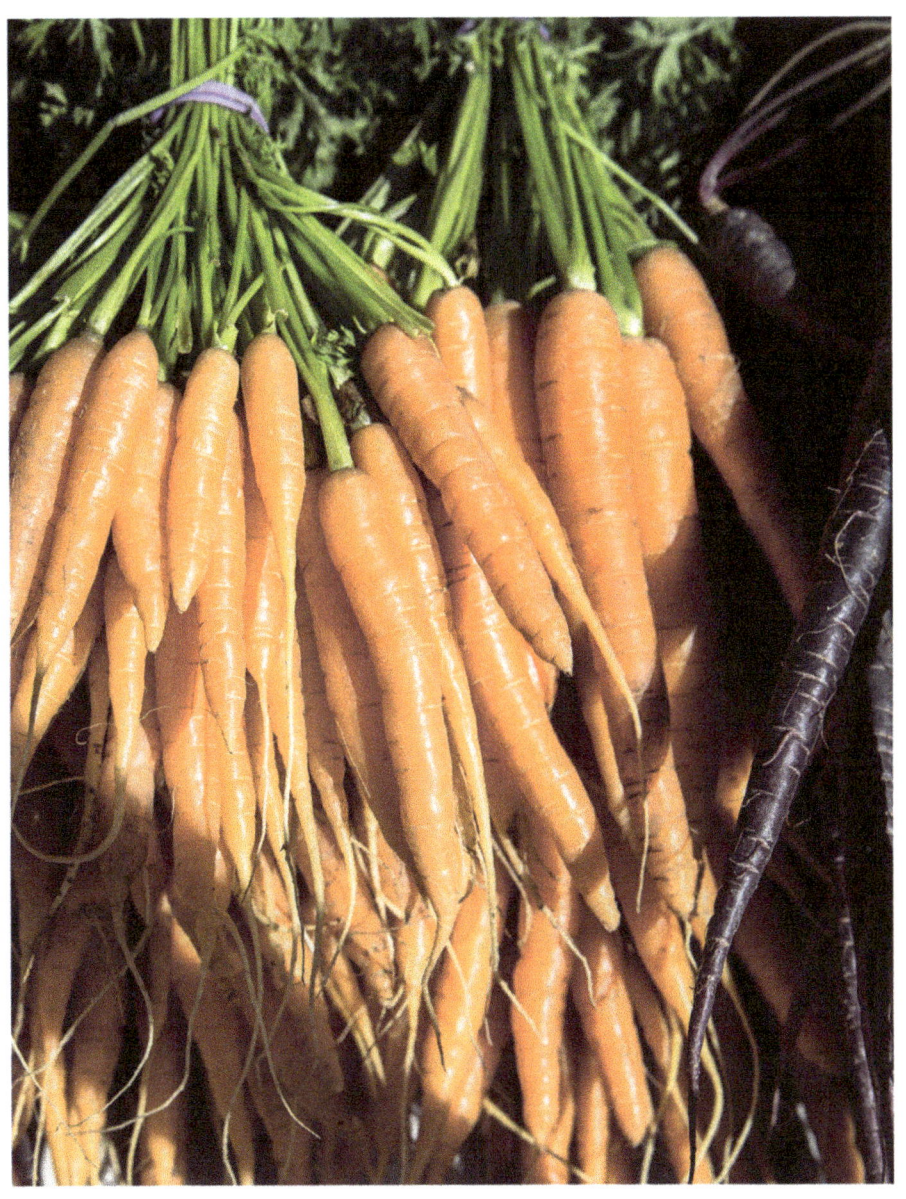

Italian Breakfast Salad

Prep Time: 10 min | **Cook Time:** 0 min | **Serve:** 4

- 1 handful kalamata olives, pitted and sliced
- 1 cup cherry tomatoes, halved
- 1½ cucumbers, sliced
- 1 red onion, chopped
- 2 tablespoons chopped oregano
- 1 tablespoon chopped mint

For the salad dressing:

- 2 tablespoons balsamic vinegar
- ¼ cup olive oil
- 1 garlic clove, minced
- 2 teaspoons dried Italian herbs
- A pinch of salt and black pepper

1.In a salad bowl, toss together the olives with the tomatoes, cucumbers, onion, mint, and oregano. In a smaller bowl, whisk the vinegar with the oil, garlic, Italian herbs, salt, and pepper. Pour the dressing over the salad, toss and serve for breakfast.

Nutrition: calories 191, fat 10, fiber 3, carbs 13, protein 1

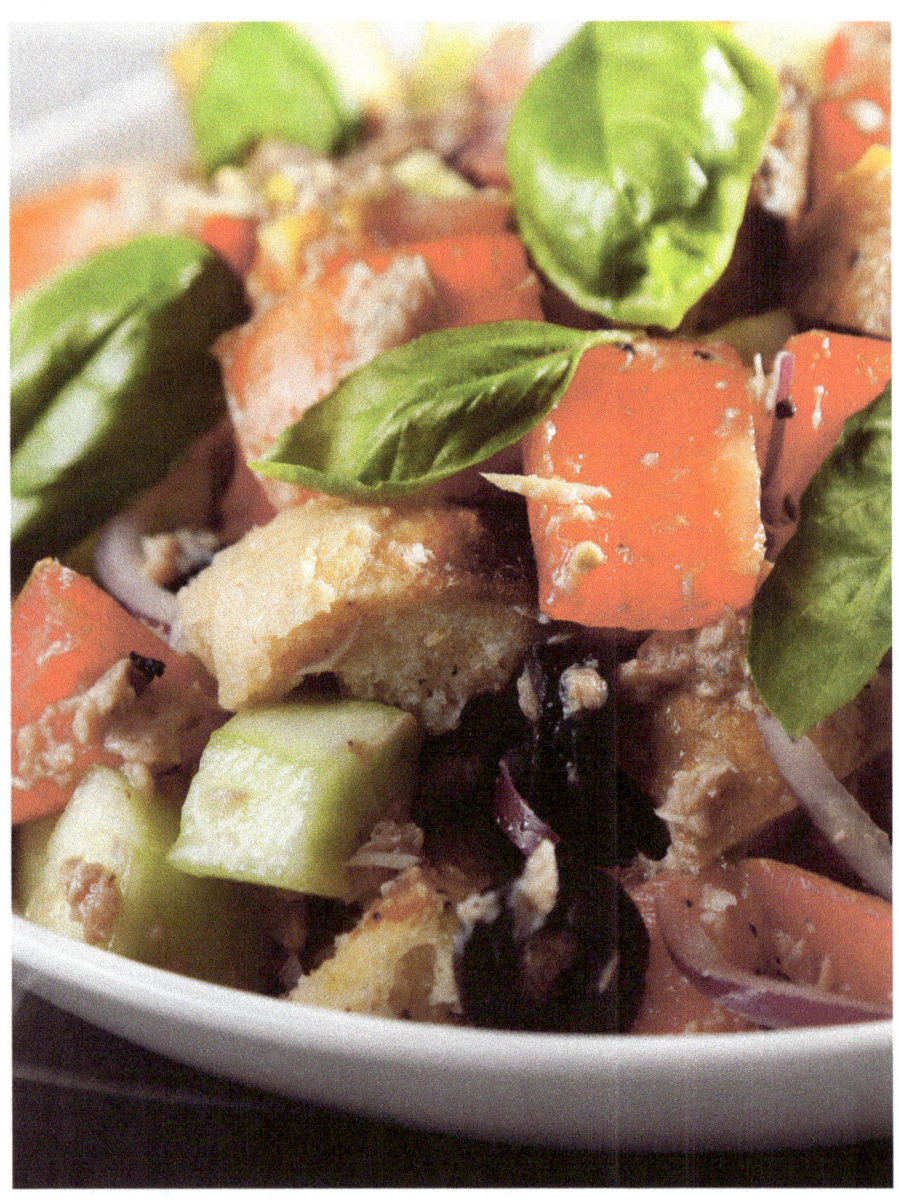

Zucchini and Sprout Breakfast Mix

Prep Time: 10 min | **Cook Time:** 0 min | **Serve:** 4

- 2 zucchinis, spiralized
- 2 cups bean sprouts
- 4 green onions, chopped
- 1 red bell pepper, chopped
- Juice of 1 lime
- 1 tablespoon olive oil
- ½ cup chopped cilantro
- ¾ cup almonds chopped
- A pinch of salt and black pepper

1.In a salad bowl, toss together the zucchinis with the bean sprouts, green onions, bell pepper, cilantro, almonds, salt, pepper, lime juice, and oil. Serve for breakfast.

Nutrition: calories 140, fat 4, fiber 2, carbs 7, protein 8 20.

Breakfast Corn Salad

Prep Time: 10 min | **Cook Time:** 0 min | **Serve:** 4

- 2 avocados, pitted, peeled, and cubed
- 1-pint mixed cherry tomatoes halved
- 2 cups fresh corn kernels
- 1 red onion, chopped

For the salad dressing:
- 2 tablespoons olive oil
- 1 tablespoon lime juice
- ½ teaspoon grated lime zest
- A pinch of salt and black pepper
- ¼ cup chopped cilantro

1.In a salad bowl, mix the avocados with tomatoes, corn, and onion. Add the oil, lime juice, lime zest, salt, pepper, and cilantro, toss and serve for breakfast.

Nutrition: calories 140, fat 3, fiber 2, carbs 6, protein 9 21.

Simple Basil Tomato Mix

Prep Time: 10 min | **Cook Time:** 0 min | **Serve:** 6

- ½ cup extra-virgin olive oil
- 1 cucumber, chopped
- 2 pints colored cherry tomatoes, halved Salt, and black pepper to the taste
- 1 red onion, chopped
- 3 tablespoons red vinegar
- 1 garlic clove, minced
- 1 bunch basil, roughly chopped

1.In a salad bowl, toss together the cucumber with the tomatoes, onion, salt, pepper, oil, vinegar, basil, and garlic.

Nutrition: calories 100, fat 1, fiber 2, carbs 2, protein 6 22.

Cucumber and Avocado Salad

Prep Time: 10 min | **Cook Time:** 0 min | **Serve:** 4

- 1-pound cucumbers, chopped
- 2 avocados, pitted and chopped
- 1 small red onion, thinly sliced
- 2 tablespoons olive oil
- 2 tablespoons lemon juice
- ¼ cup chopped parsley
- A pinch of salt and black pepper

1.In a salad bowl, mix the cucumbers with the avocados, onion, oil, lemon juice, parsley, salt, and pepper. Serve for breakfast.

Nutrition: calories 120, fat 2, fiber 2, carbs 3, protein 4

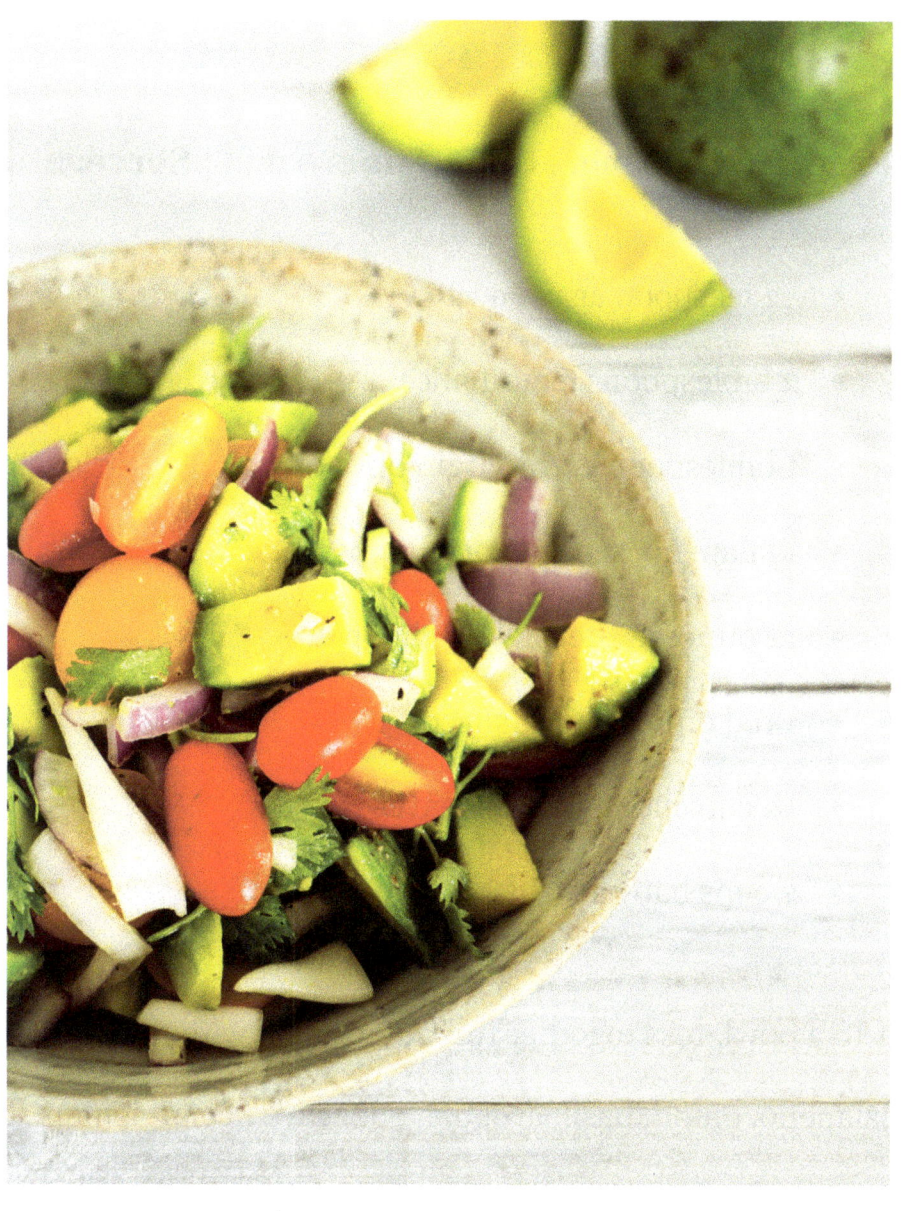

Watermelon Salad

Prep Time: 10 min | **Cook Time**: 0 min | **Serve**: 2

- ½ teaspoon agave nectar
- 2 tablespoons lemon juice
- 1 tablespoon extra-virgin olive oil
- 1 jalapeno, seeded and chopped
- 12 ounces watermelon, chopped
- 1 red onion, thinly sliced
- ½ cup chopped basil leaves
- 2 cups baby arugula

1.In a bowl, toss together the watermelon with the jalapeno, onion, basil, arugula, oil, agave nectar, lemon juice, and oil.

Nutrition: calories 128, fat 8, fiber 2, carbs 16, protein 2

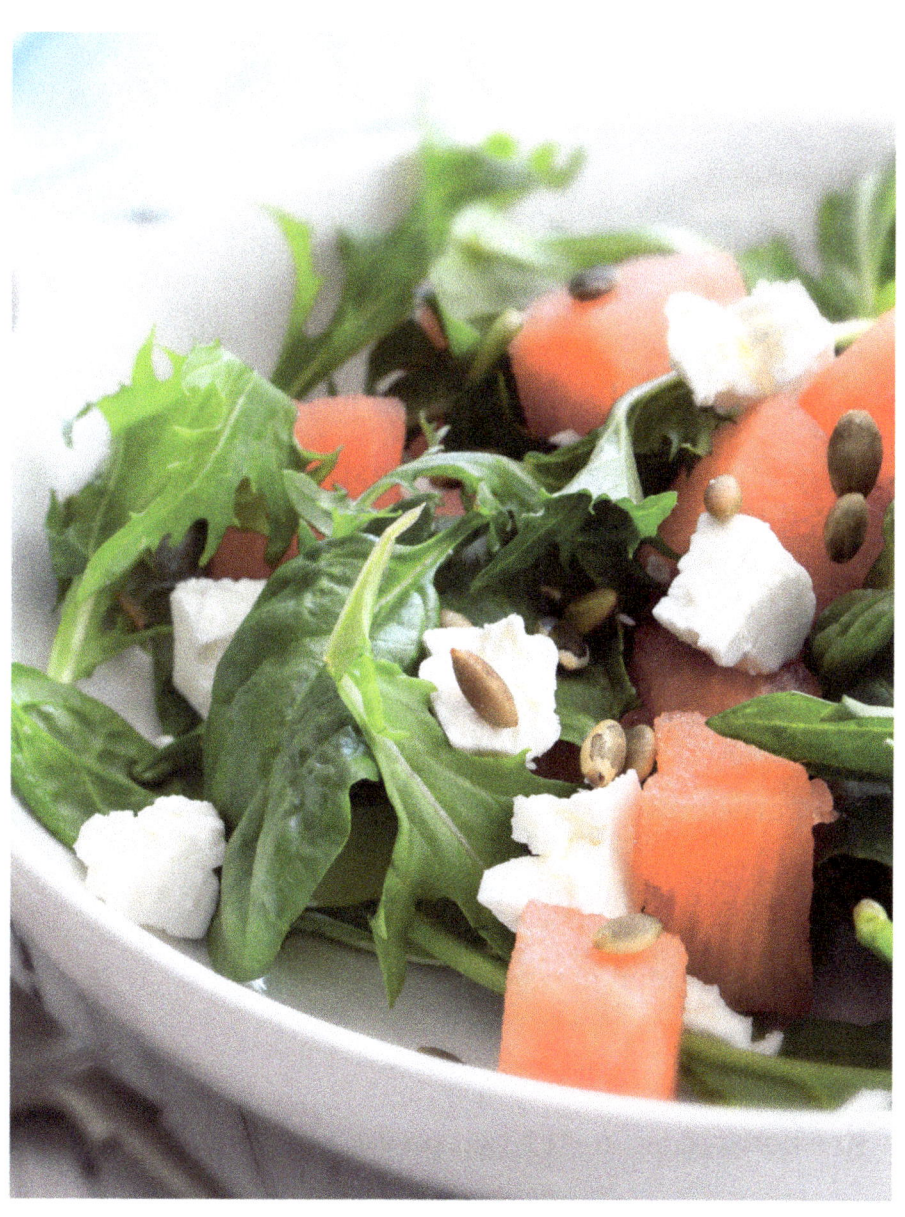

Peppers and Olives Salad

Prep Time: 10 min | **Cook Time:** 0 min | **Serve:** 4

- 1 red bell pepper, cut into strips
- 1 green bell pepper, cut into strips
- 2 spring onions, chopped
- 1 cup black olives, pitted and halved
- 1 cup kalamata olives, pitted and halved A pinch of garlic powder
- A pinch of salt and black pepper
- 1 tablespoon avocado oil

1.In a bowl, combine the bell peppers with the onions and the other ingredients, toss, divide between plates, and serve breakfast.

Nutrition: calories 221, fat 6, fiber 6, carbs 14, protein 11

Sweet Potato, Spinach, and Eggs Mix

Prep Time: 5 min | **Cook Time:** 15 min | **Serve:** 4

- A pinch of salt and black pepper
- 8 eggs, whisked
- 1 tablespoon olive oil
- 1 small yellow onion, chopped
- 2 garlic cloves, minced
- 1 cup sweet potato, peeled, and cup bed
- 1 cup baby spinach
- 1 tablespoon chives, chopped

1. Heat a pan with the oil over medium-high heat, add the onion and the garlic and sauté for 2 minutes.

2. Add the potato, stir and cook for 3 minutes more.

3.Add the eggs and the other ingredients, cook for 10 minutes, stirring from time to time, divide between plates, and serve breakfast.

Nutrition: calories 213.3, fat 12.3, fiber 7, carbs 14, protein 2.3

Avocado and Mango Salad

Prep Time: 5 min | **Cook Time:** 0 min | **Serve:** 2

- 2 avocados, peeled, pitted, and roughly cubed
- 1 mango, peeled and cubed
- 1 tablespoon lime juice
- 1 cup baby spinach
- Handful basil, torn
- 1 tablespoon olive oil
- ¼ cup pine nuts, toasted
- A pinch of salt and black pepper

1. In a salad bowl, mix avocados with the mango and the other ingredients, toss and serve for breakfast.

Nutrition: calories 200.1, fat 4, fiber 4, carbs 14.1, protein 5

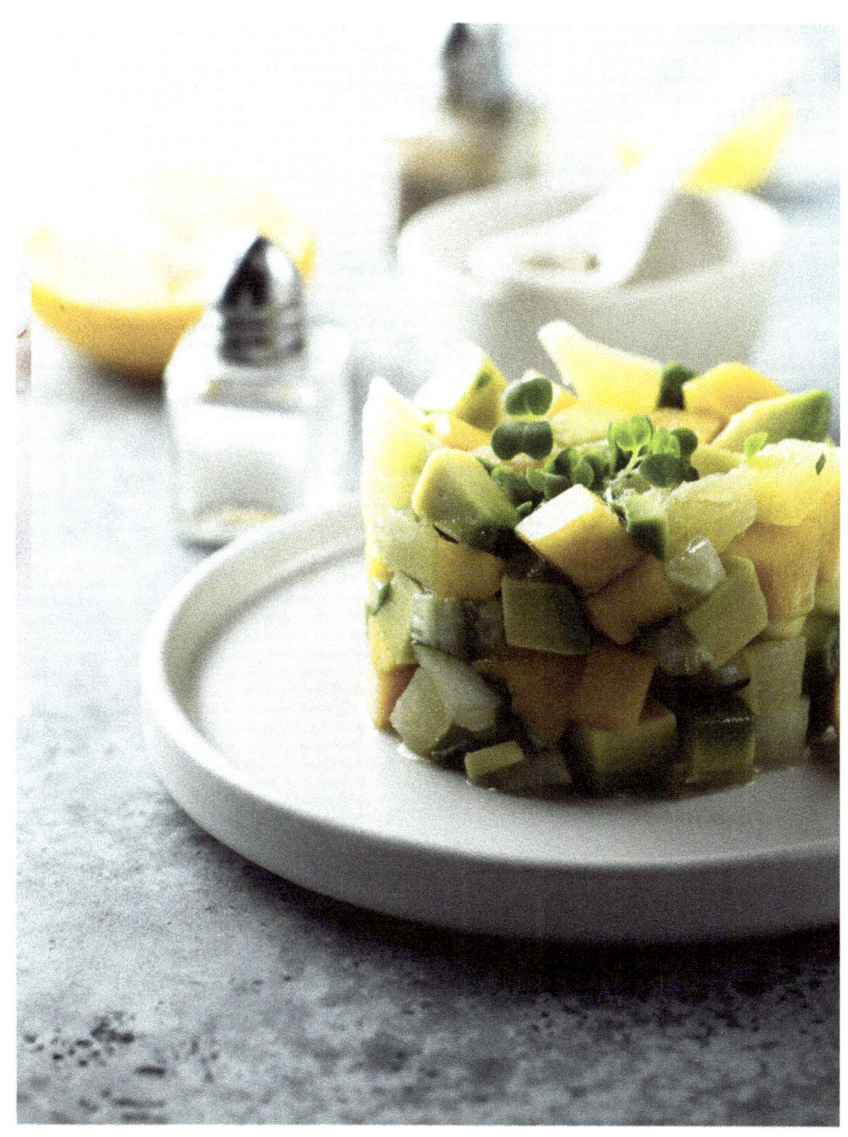

Brussels Sprouts Eggs with Turmeric

Prep Time: 10 min | **Cook Time:** 15 min | **Serve:** 4

- 1 cup Brussels sprouts, shredded
- 1 yellow onion, chopped
- 8 eggs, whisked
- 1 tablespoon olive oil
- 1 tablespoon turmeric powder
- 1 tablespoon cilantro, chopped
- 1 teaspoon cumin, ground
- A pinch of salt and black pepper

1.Heat a pan with the oil over medium-high heat, add the onion and the sprouts and sauté for 5 minutes.

2.Add the eggs and the other ingredients, toss well, cook for 10 minutes more, divide between plates and serve.

Nutrition: calories 177, fat 2, fiber 6, carbs 15, protein 6

Strawberries and Spinach Bowls

Prep Time: 5 min | **Cook Time:** 0 min | **Serve:** 4

- 2 cups baby spinach
- 10 strawberries, halved
- 1 tablespoon pine nuts
- 1 tablespoon almonds, chopped
- 1 tablespoon lime juice
- 1 tablespoon avocado oil

1.In a bowl, combine the spinach with the strawberries and the other ingredients, toss and serve for breakfast.

Nutrition: calories 171, fat 3, fiber 6, carbs 15, protein 5

Collard and Spinach Oatmeal

Prep Time: 10 min | **Cook Time:** 20 min | **Serve:** 4

- 1 cup old-fashioned oats
- 1 cup almond milk
- ½ cup water
- 1 tablespoon coconut oil, melted
- ½ cup collard greens, chopped
- ½ cup baby spinach, chopped
- A handful basil, chopped
- ½ tablespoon rosemary, chopped
- A pinch of salt and black pepper

1.Heat a pot with the milk and the water over medium heat, add the oats, the oil, and the other ingredients, cook for 20 minutes, stirring often, divide into bowls and serve warm.

Nutrition: calories 246, fat 19.3, fiber 3.8, carbs 17.6, protein 4.1

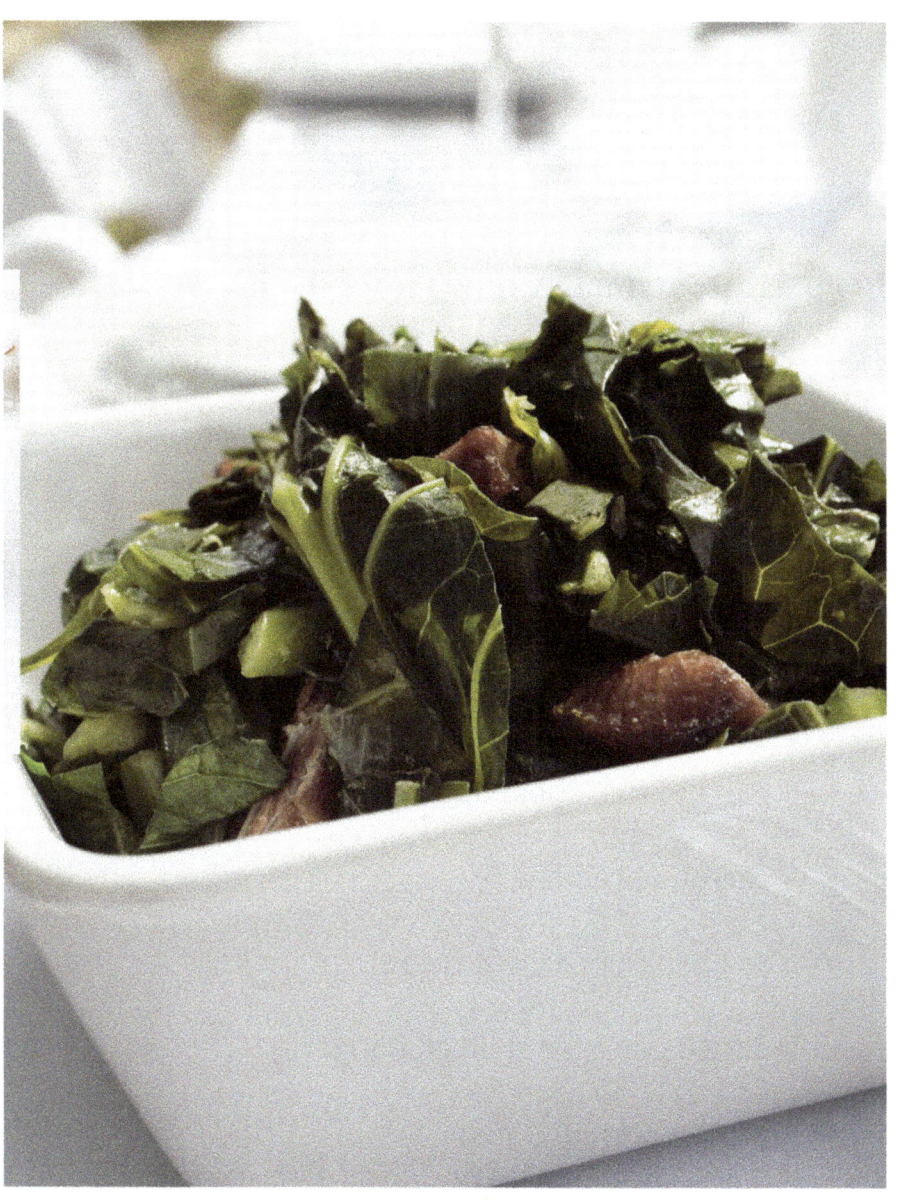

Spinach, Kale and Quinoa Salad

Prep Time: 10 min | **Cook Time:** 0 min | **Serve:** 4

- 1 cup baby spinach
- 1 cup baby kale
- 2 spring onions, chopped
- 2 tablespoons olive oil
- 1 cup quinoa, cooked
- 1 carrot, shredded
- 1 red bell pepper, cut into strips
- A pinch of salt and black pepper
- 1 tablespoon lime juice
- 4 eggs, hard boiled, peeled and roughly cubed

1.In a salad bowl, combine the quinoa with the spinach, kale and the other ingredients, toss and serve for breakfast.

Nutrition: calories 308, fat 14.1, fiber 4.4, carbs 34, protein 12.8

Fennel, Kale and Barley Salad

Prep Time: 10 min | **Cook Time:** 1 hour | **Serve:** 2

- 1 cup black barley
- 3 cups water
- 2 fennel bulbs, shaved
- 1 cup baby kale
- 1 small red onion, sliced
- 2 tablespoons almonds, chopped
- 1 avocado, peeled, pitted, and cubed
- 2 tablespoons oil
- 1 tablespoon pine nuts
- 2 tablespoons balsamic vinegar
- A pinch of salt and black pepper

1.Put the barley in a pot, add the water, salt, and pepper, bring to a simmer over medium heat, cook for 1 hour, drain, cool and transfer to a salad bowl.

2.Add the fennel, kale, and the other ingredients, toss, divide into smaller bowls, and serve for breakfast.

Nutrition: calories 545, fat 41.2, fiber 18.1, carbs 42.7, protein 9.8

Chili Carrot and Sweet Potato Mix

Prep Time: 5 min | **Cook Time:** 20 min | **Serve:** 4

- 2 scallions, chopped
- 2 tablespoons olive oil
- 4 sweet potatoes, peeled and cut into wedges
- 1 teaspoon chili powder
- 1 teaspoon hot paprika
- 2 carrots, shredded
- 1 teaspoon sesame seeds
- 1 tablespoon lime juice
- A pinch of salt and black pepper

1.Heat a pan with the oil over medium heat, add the scallions and sauté for 2 minutes.

2.Add the sweet potatoes and the other ingredients, toss, cook for 18 minutes more, divide into bowls and serve for breakfast.

Nutrition: calories 371, fat 12.2, fiber 6, carbs 13.1, protein 5

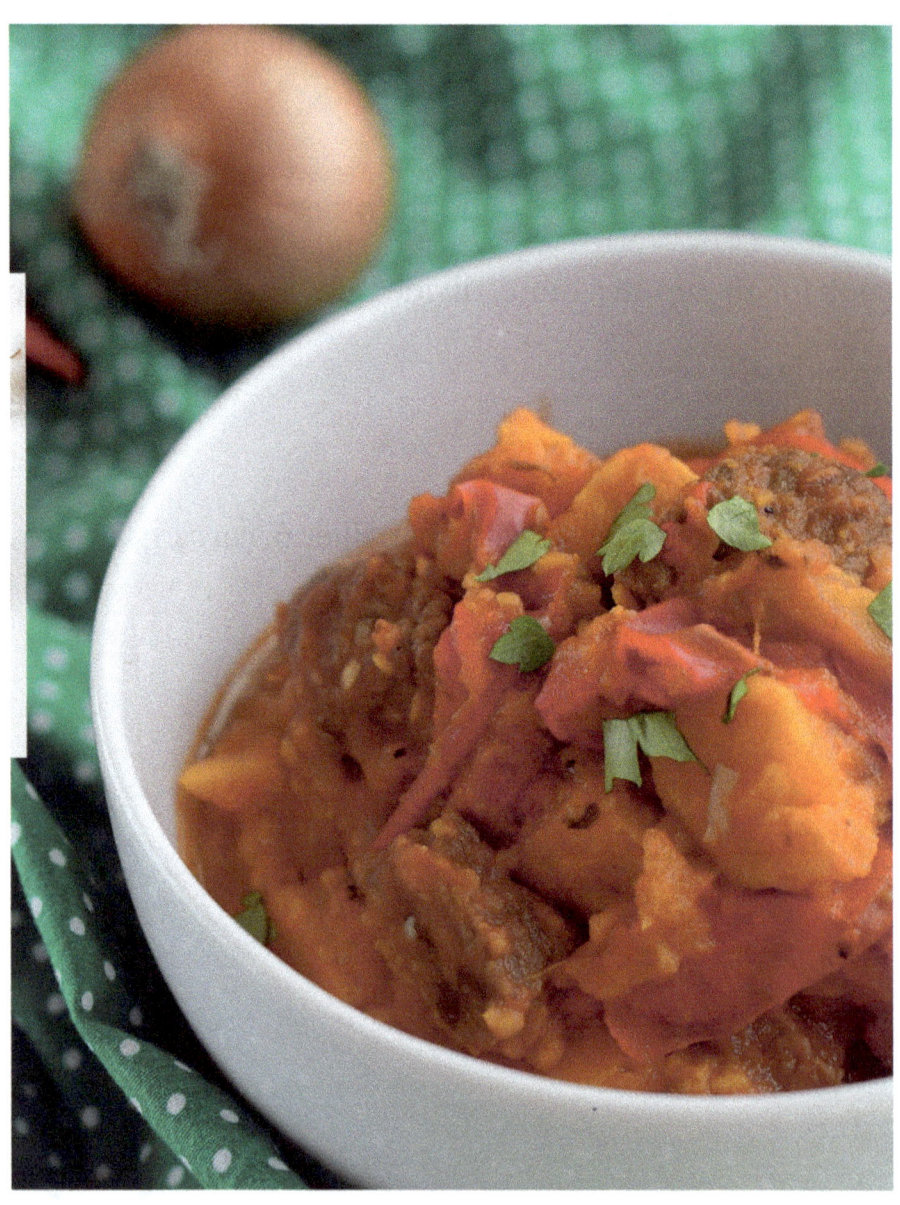

Jalapeno Cucumber Bowls

Prep Time: 5 min | **Cook Time:** 0 min | **Serve:** 4

- 2 tablespoons olive oil
- 2 scallions, chopped
- 1 tablespoon lime juice
- 1 tablespoon dill, chopped
- 3 cucumbers, roughly cubed
- 2 tablespoons chives, chopped
- 1 jalapeno, chopped
- Handful basil, chopped
- 1 tablespoon almonds, crushed
- 1 tablespoon walnuts, chopped
- A pinch of salt and black pepper

1.In a salad bowl, combine the cucumbers with the scallions and the other ingredients, toss, divide into smaller bowls, and serve breakfast.

Nutrition: calories 199, fat 4, fiber 8, carbs 15, protein 4

Zucchinis, Arugula, and Barley Mix

Prep Time: 10 min | **Cook Time:** 0 min | **Serve:** 4

- 2 zucchinis, cut with a spiralizer
- 1 cup barley, cooked
- 2 scallions, chopped
- 1 tablespoon olive oil
- ½ teaspoon sweet paprika
- A pinch of chili powder
- 1 tablespoon lime juice
- A pinch of salt and black pepper
- 1 tablespoon oregano, chopped
- 2 cups baby arugula
- ½ cup sesame seeds paste

- 1 tablespoon balsamic vinegar
- 1 garlic clove, minced
- ½ teaspoon cumin, ground

1.In a large bowl, combine the zucchinis with the barley, scallions, and the other ingredients, toss, divide between plates, and serve breakfast.

Nutrition: calories 226, fat 5, fiber 7, carbs 16, protein 7

Avocado and Pepper Eggs Mix

Prep Time: 10 min | **Cook Time:** 15 min | **Serve:** 4

- 1 avocado, peeled, pitted, and cubed
- 8 eggs, whisked
- 2 scallions, chopped
- 1 red bell pepper, chopped
- 2 tablespoons olive oil
- 2 garlic cloves, minced
- 1 tablespoon cilantro, chopped

1.Heat a pan with the oil over medium-high heat, add the scallions, garlic, bell pepper, and sauté for 5 minutes.

2.Add the avocado and the other ingredients, toss, cook for 10 minutes over medium heat, divide between plates and serve.

Nutrition: calories 211, fat 2, fiber 5, carbs 16, protein 5

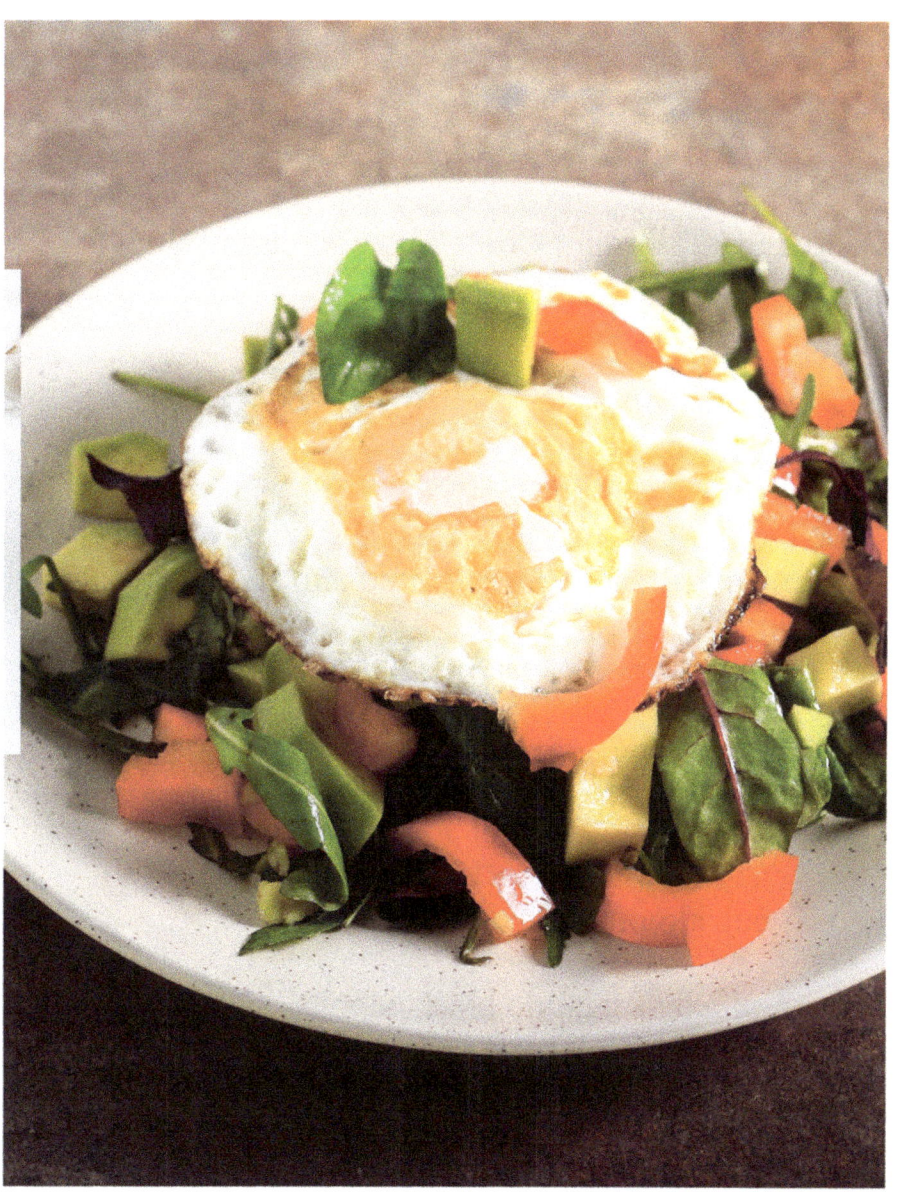

Olives Frittata with Shallots

Prep Time: 10 min | **Cook Time:** 20 min | **Serve:** 4

- 8 eggs, whisked
- 2 shallots, chopped
- 1 cup kalamata olives, pitted and chopped
- 1 tablespoon coriander, chopped
- 1 tablespoon chives, chopped
- 1 tablespoon olive oil
- 1 cup almond milk
- A pinch of salt and black pepper

1. Heat a pan with the oil over medium heat, add the shallots and sauté for 2 minutes.

2.Add the eggs mixed with the milk and the other ingredients, toss, spread into the pan, introduce the frittata in the oven and cook at 360 degrees F for 18 minutes.

3.Divide the frittata between plates and serve.

Nutrition: calories 201, fat 6, fiber 9, carbs 14, protein 6

Berries Coconut Mix

Prep Time: 10 min | **Cook Time:** 15 min | **Serve:** 4

- 1 cup blueberries
- 1 tablespoon coconut oil, melted
- 1/3 cup coconut flakes
- 1 cup coconut milk
- ½ teaspoon nutmeg, ground
- ½ teaspoon vanilla extract

1.In a small pot, mix the berries with the oil and the other ingredients, toss, simmer over medium heat for 15 minutes, divide into bowls and serve.

Nutrition: calories 208, fat 2, fiber 6, carbs 16, protein 8

Cucumber, Spinach, and Olives Salad

Prep Time: 5 min | **Cook Time:** 0 min | **Serve:** 4

- 2 cups baby spinach, torn
- 2 shallots, chopped
- 1 cup cucumber, cubed
- 1 cup kalamata olives, pitted and sliced
- 1 tablespoon chives, chopped
- 1 tablespoon balsamic vinegar
- A pinch of salt and black pepper
- 2 tablespoons olive oil

1.In a salad bowl, mix the spinach with the shallots, the cucumber, and the other ingredients, toss, divide between plates, and serve breakfast.

Nutrition: calories 171, fat 2, fiber 5, carbs 11, protein 5

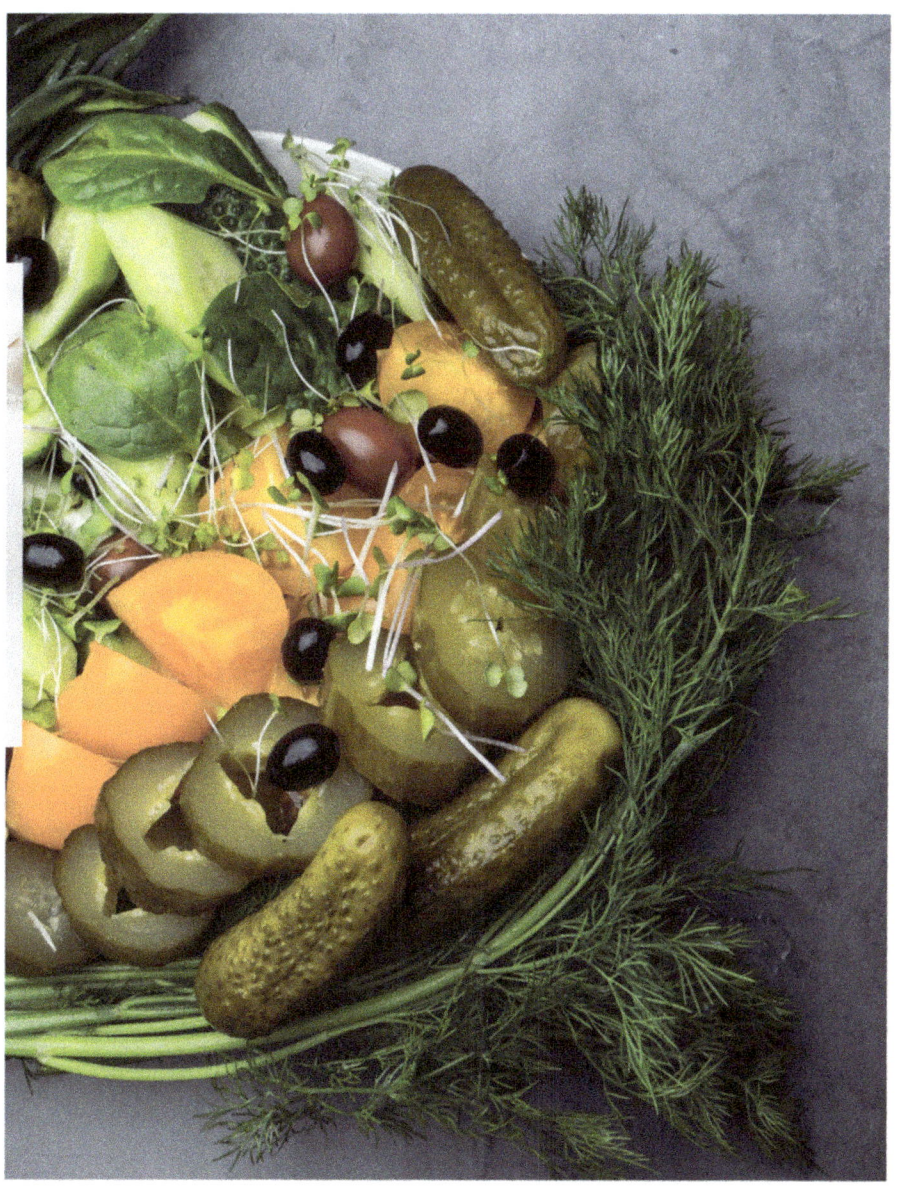

Sweet Potato Bowls

Prep Time: 5 min | **Cook Time:** 20 min | **Serve:** 4

- 2 sweet potatoes, peeled and cubed
- 1 cup coconut cream
- 3 garlic cloves, minced
- 2 tablespoons olive oil
- 1 yellow onion, chopped
- 1 teaspoon cumin, ground
- 1 teaspoon turmeric powder
- 2 tablespoons parsley, chopped
- A pinch of salt and black pepper

1.Heat a pan with the oil over medium-high heat, add the onion, garlic, cumin, turmeric, stir and sauté for 5 minutes.

2.Add the potatoes and the other ingredients, toss, cook for 15 minutes more, divide into bowls and serve for breakfast.

Nutrition: calories 188, fat 2, fiber 8, carbs 10, protein 4

Shallots Cucumber Omelet

Prep Time: 10 min | **Cook Time:** 12 min | **Serve:** 4

- 8 eggs, whisked
- 2 shallots, chopped
- A pinch of salt and black pepper
- 1 cucumber, cubed
- 1 tablespoon parsley, chopped
- 1 tablespoon olive oil

1. Heat a pan with the oil over medium-high heat, add the shallots and sauté for 2 minutes.
2. Add the eggs mixed with the other ingredients, toss, spread into the pan, cook for 5 minutes, flip and cook for another 5 minutes.

3.Cut the omelet, divide it between plates and serve for breakfast.

Nutrition: calories 201, fat 2, fiber 5, carbs 11, protein 5

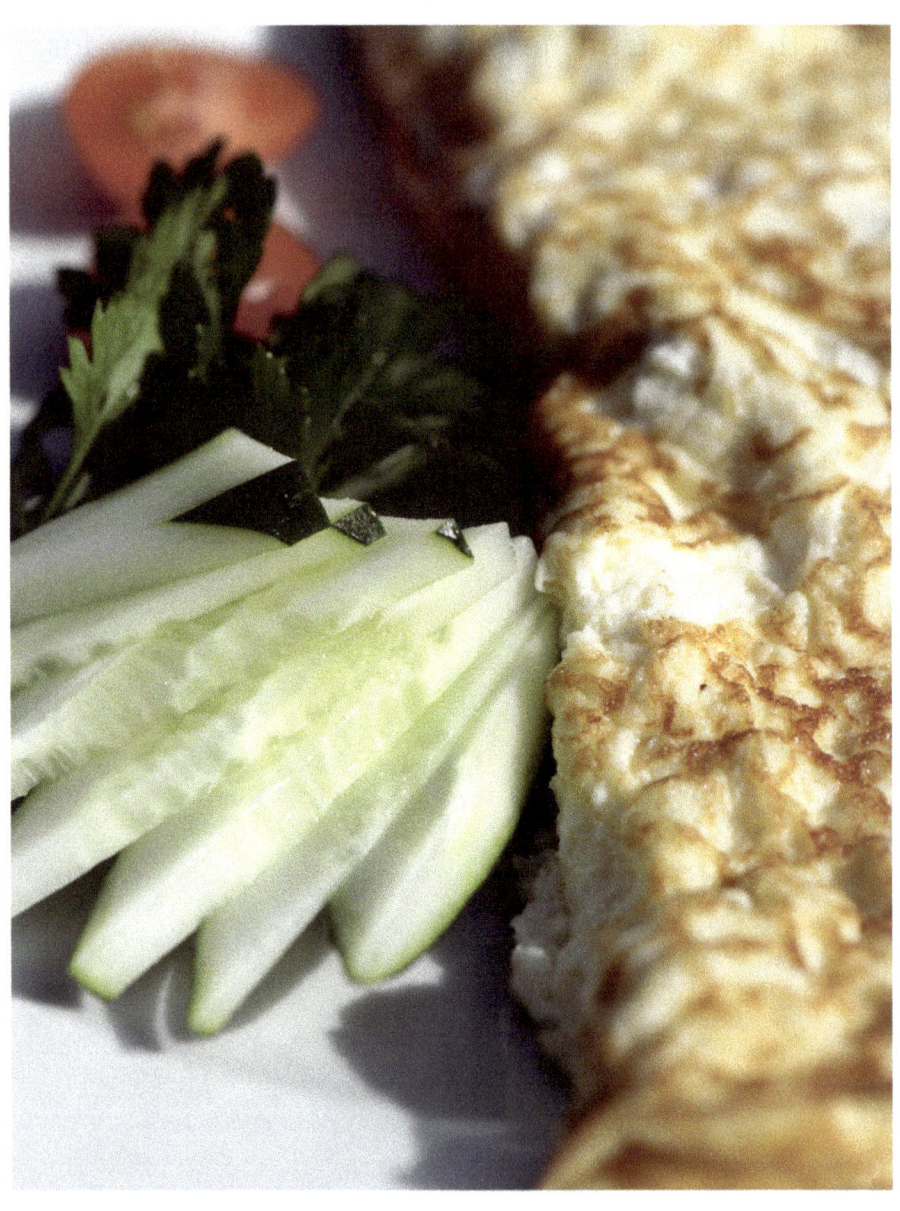

Cinnamon Oatmeal with Maple Syrup

Prep Time: 10 min | **Cook Time:** 20 min | **Serve:** 4

- 2 cups coconut milk
- 1 cup old fashioned oats
- 2 tablespoons flax meal
- 1 teaspoon vanilla extract
- 2 teaspoons cinnamon powder
- 1 teaspoon maple syrup

1.In a small pot, mix the oats with the milk and the other ingredients, toss, bring to a simmer, cook over medium heat for 20 minutes, divide into bowls and serve for breakfast.

Nutrition: calories 454, fat 32.4, fiber 7.6, carbs 35.7, protein 8.5

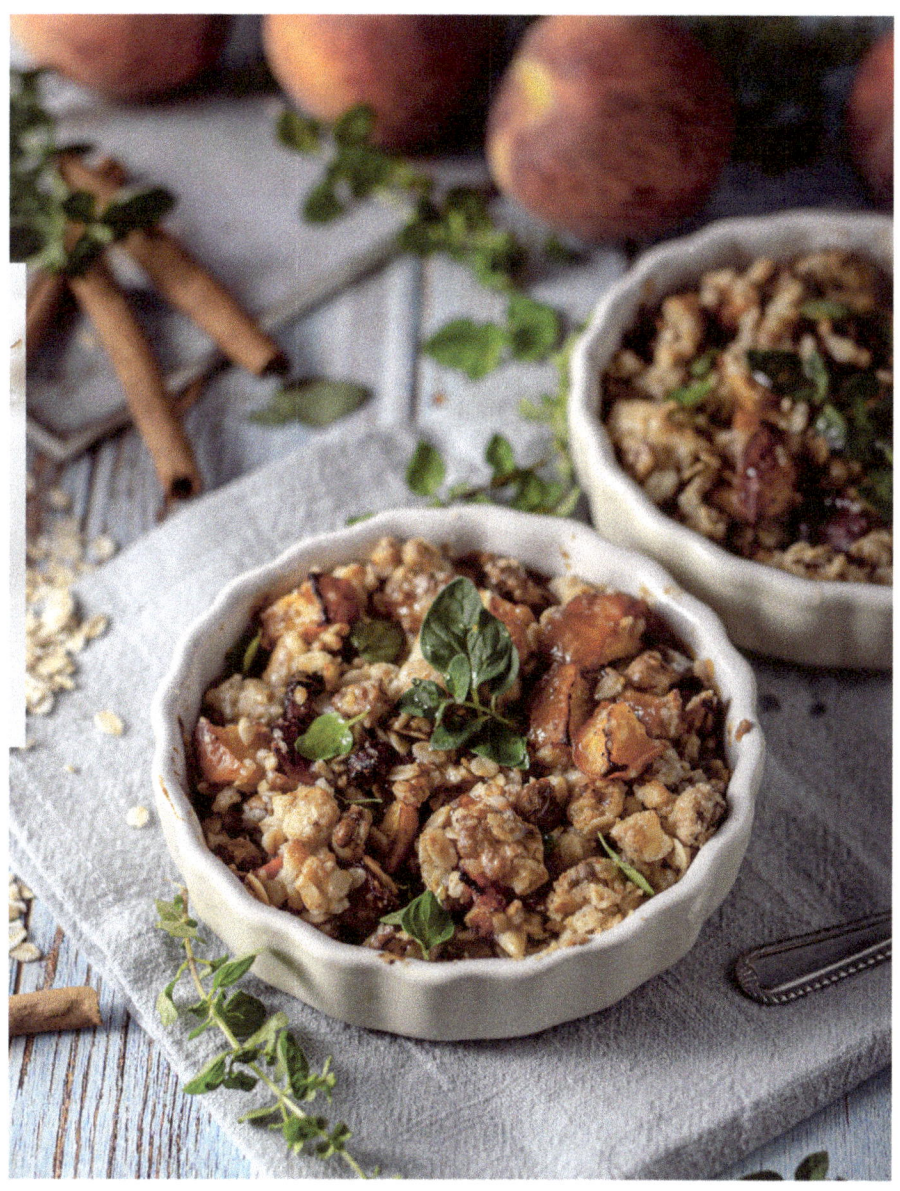

Chili Broccoli Salad

Prep Time: 10 min | **Cook Time:** 15 min | **Serve:** 4

- 1 pound broccoli florets
- 1 yellow onion, chopped
- 1 tablespoon olive oil
- ½ cup coconut cream
- 1 teaspoon chili powder
- 1 teaspoon hot paprika
- 1 teaspoon garlic powder
- A pinch of salt and black pepper

1. Heat a pan with the oil over medium-high heat, add the onion and sauté for 2 minutes.

2.Add the rest of the ingredients, toss, cook for 12 minutes over medium heat, divide into bowls, and serve breakfast.

Nutrition: calories 153, fat 11.2, fiber 4.5, carbs 12.7, protein 4.4

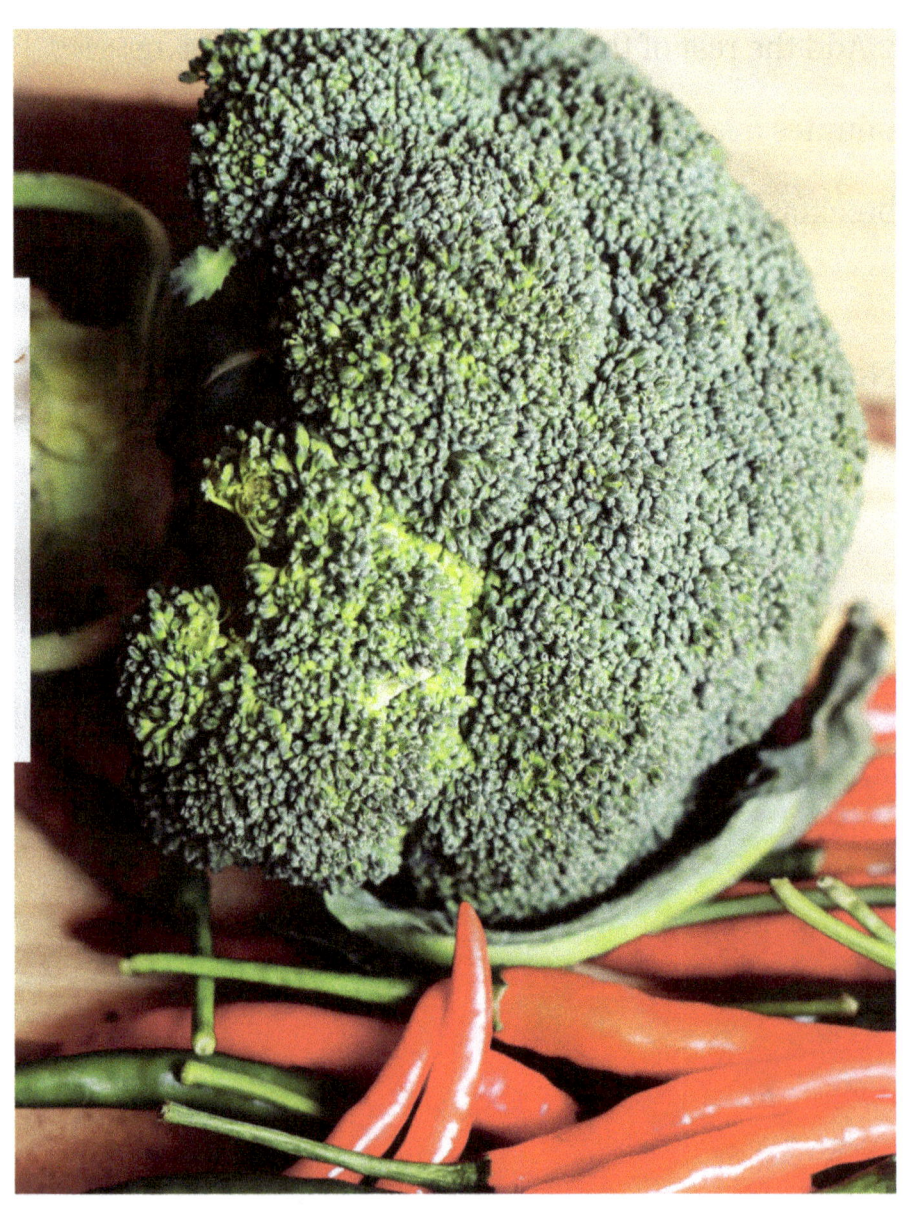

Spinach, Kale, and Olives Bowls

Prep Time: 5 min | **Cook Time:** 0 min | **Serve:** 4

- 1 cup spinach, torn
- 1 cup kale, torn
- 1 cup black olives, pitted and halved
- 2 shallots, chopped
- 1 tablespoon lemon juice
- 1 tablespoon avocado oil
- 1 tablespoon mint, chopped

1. In a bowl, mix the spinach with the kale and the other ingredients, toss, and serve breakfast.

Nutrition: calories 198, fat 6.4, fiber 2, carbs 8, protein 6

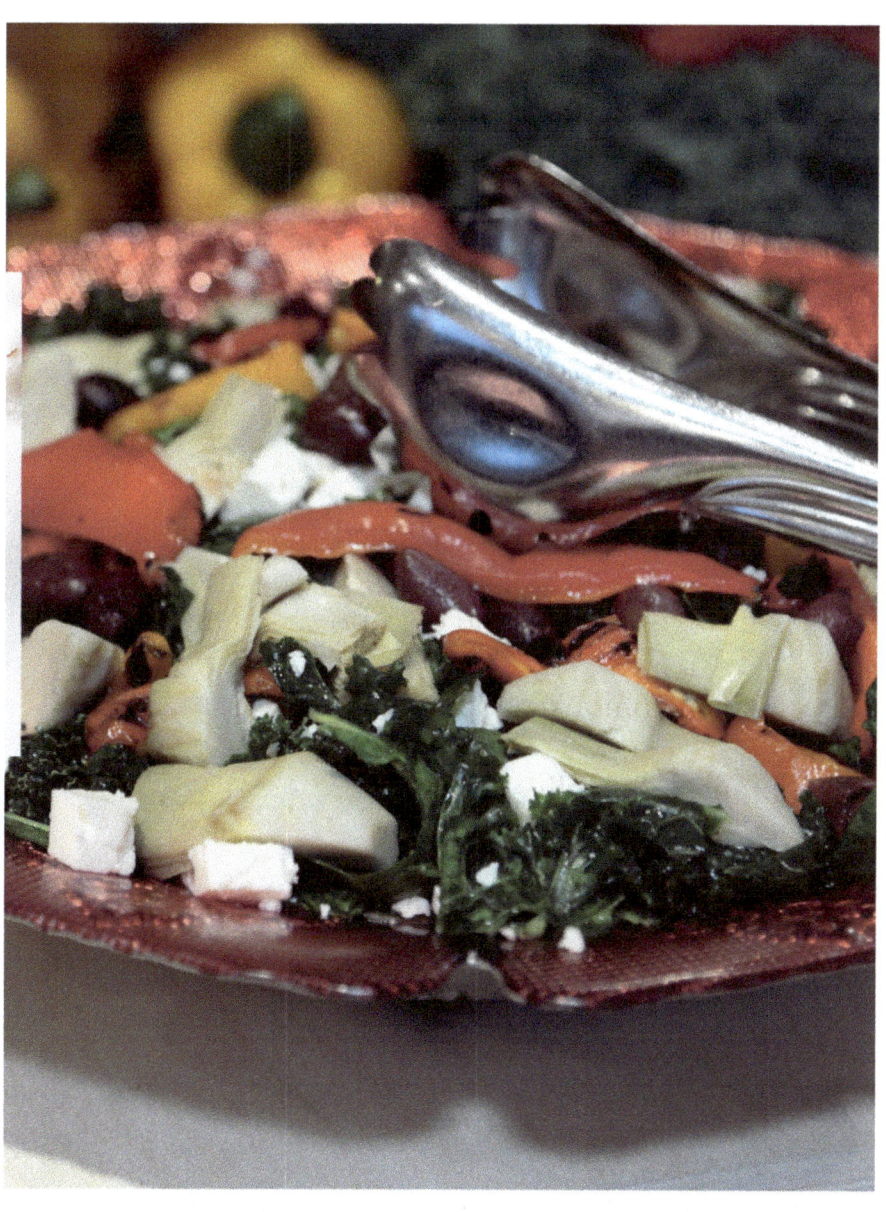

Cherry Tomato and Orange Salad

Prep Time: 6 min | **Cook Time:** 0 min | **Serve:** 4

- 1 cup cherry tomatoes, halved
- 2 oranges, peeled and cut into segments
- 3 spring onions, chopped
- 1 tablespoon olive oil
- 1 tablespoon lemon juice
- A pinch of salt and black pepper
- 1 teaspoon turmeric powder

1. In a bowl, mix the tomatoes with the oranges and the other ingredients, toss, and serve breakfast.

Nutrition: calories 255, fat 4, fiber 5, carbs 15, protein 6

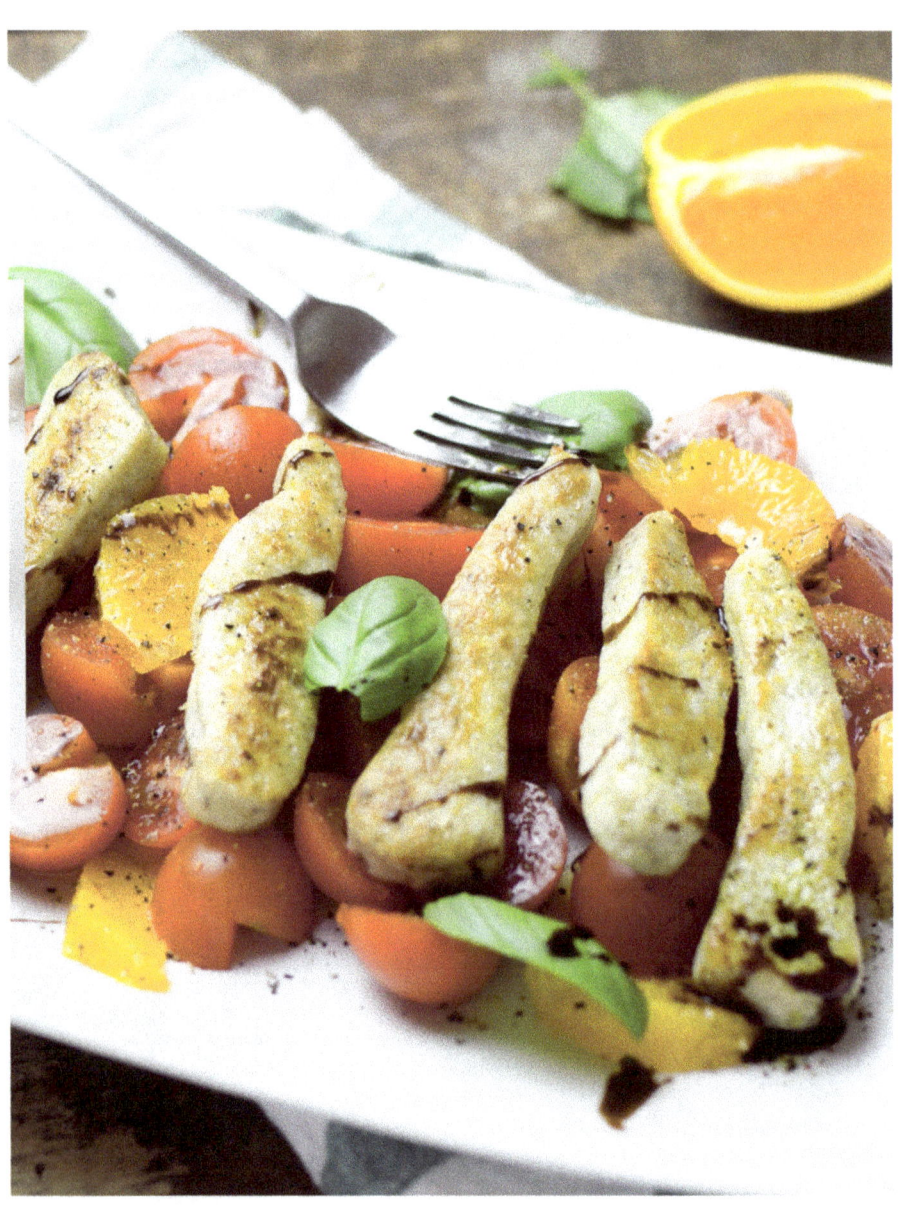

Pear and Kale Salad

Prep Time: 10 min | **Cook Time:** 15 min | **Serve:** 4

- 2 cups pears, cored and cubed
- 1/3 cup coconut flakes, unsweetened
- 2 tablespoons orange juice
- 1 cup baby kale
- 1 tablespoon avocado oil

1.In a bowl, combine the pears with the coconut and the other ingredients, toss and serve for breakfast.

Nutrition: calories 172, fat 5, fiber 7, carbs 8, protein 4

Berries and Cantaloupe Salad

Prep Time: 5 min | **Cook Time:** 0 min | **Serve:** 2

- 2 tablespoons walnuts, chopped
- 1 cup blackberries
- 1 cup cantaloupe, peeled and cubed
- 1 tablespoon lime juice
- 1 tablespoon orange juice
- 1 teaspoon vanilla extract

1. In a bowl, mix the blackberries with the walnuts and other ingredients, toss, divide into smaller bowls, and serve breakfast.

Nutrition: calories 90, fat 0.3, fiber 1, carbs 0, protein 5

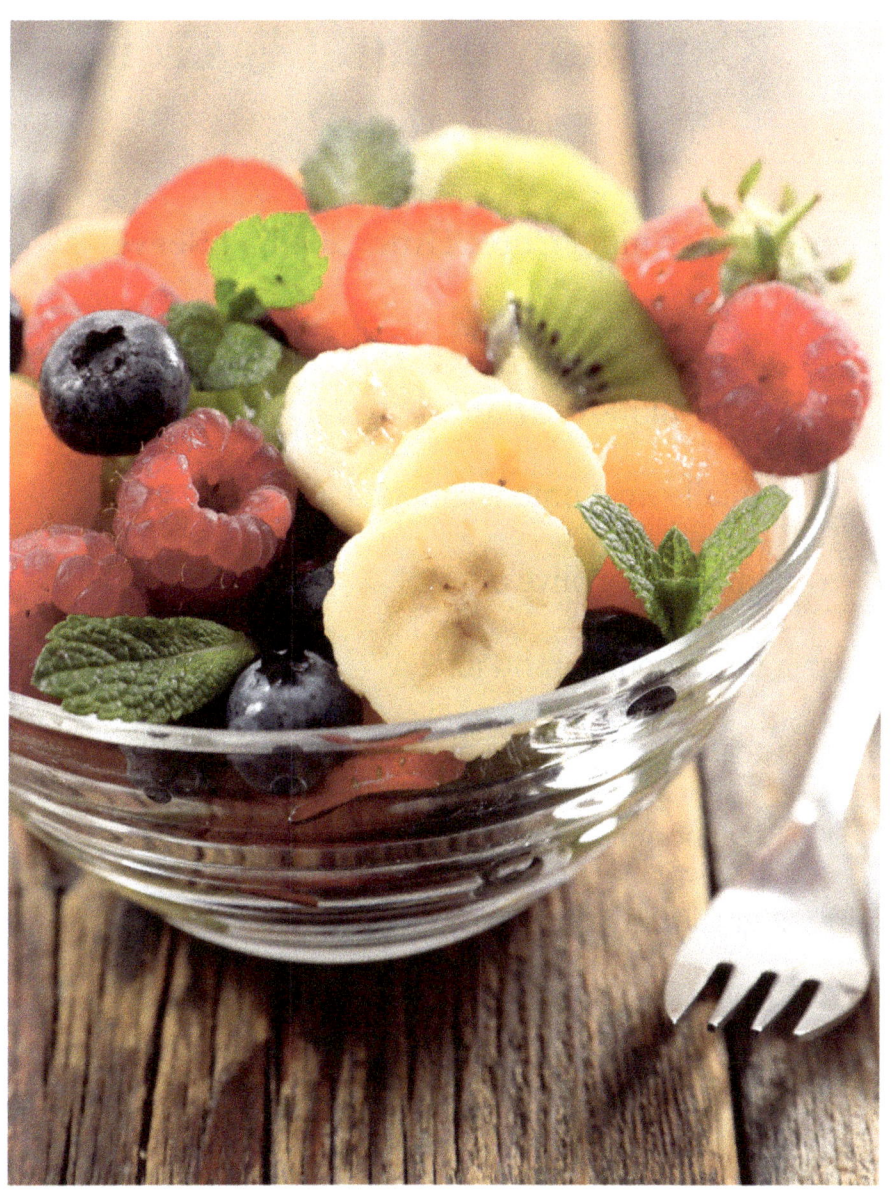

Cauliflower and Eggs Mix

Prep Time: 5 min | **Cook Time:** 20 min | **Serve:** 4

- 1 cup cauliflower florets
- 1 small sweet onion, chopped
- 1 tablespoon olive oil
- 1 tablespoon lemon juice
- 1 teaspoon turmeric powder
- 1 teaspoon cumin, ground
- 2 garlic cloves, minced
- Salt and black pepper to the taste
- 4 eggs

1.Heat a pan with the oil over medium-high heat, add the onion, and the garlic, stir and sauté for 5 minutes.

2.Add the cauliflower and cook for 5 minutes more.

3.Add the rest of the ingredients, toss, cook for 10 minutes more, divide into bowls and serve.

Nutrition: calories 214, fat 7, fiber 2, carbs 12, protein 8

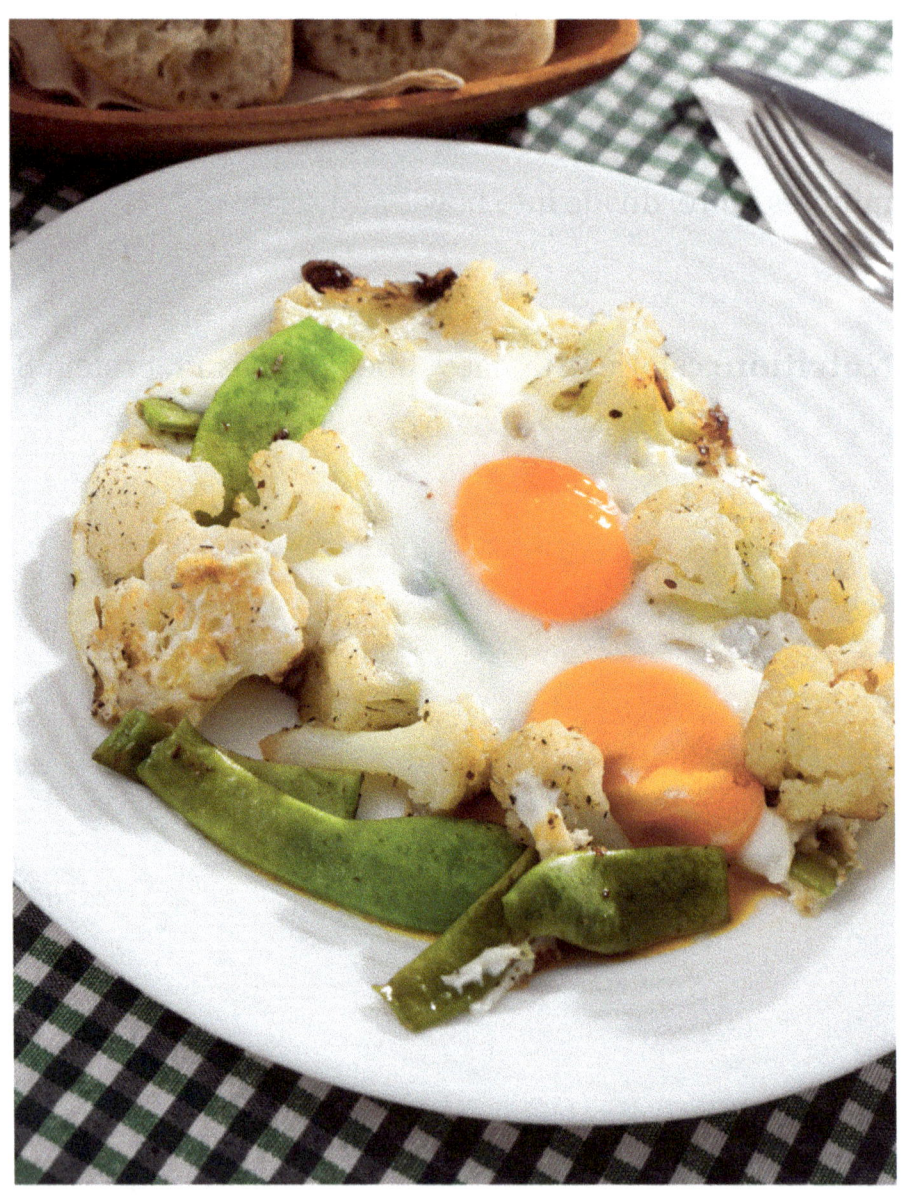

www.ingramcontent.com/pod-product-compliance
Lightning Source LLC
Chambersburg PA
CBHW070725030426
42336CB00013B/1919